EMDR and
The Art of Attunement

Esta Porter & Cindi Saj

Disclaimer: The information contained in this book is intended for licensed mental health therapists. Therapists should evaluate whether the information presented in this book is appropriate for their unique and individual client. All information presented should be used at the reader's discretion and is their sole responsibility.

ISBN:
Ebook: 979-8-89669-280-5
Paperback: 979-8-89669-324-6
Audiobook: 979-8-89669-283-6

First Edition

Table of Contents

Acknowledgment

As we embark on this journey of exploring EMDR *and the Art of Attunement*, we extend our deepest gratitude to the individuals who have shaped our paths, both personally, professionally, and spiritually.

To our families and friends: thank you for your unwavering support, encouragement, and patience. Your belief in our work gave us the space to create this book.

To our mentors and colleagues: we are profoundly grateful for the wisdom you have shared, the questions you have raised, and the rich dialogue that has kept our thinking sharp and our hearts open. The field of EMDR continues to evolve because of your collective contributions.

To our clients: your courage, vulnerability, and trust have been our greatest teachers. It is an honor to walk beside you in the healing process. You have shown us what attunement truly means—not just as a clinical skill, but as a deeply human art.

To all EMDR practitioners and seekers of therapeutic excellence: This book is dedicated to your ongoing journey of therapeutic excellence. May it serve not as a manual of answers, but as a companion in your pursuit of attuned, ethical, and compassionate care.

Finally, we humbly and respectfully acknowledge that we live, work, play, and practice on the ancestral lands of the First Nations, Métis, and Inuit peoples, who have held and protected these territories since time immemorial. Their enduring presence and wisdom continue to inspire our commitment to culturally grounded and trauma-informed healing.

We know what we know, and more importantly, we know that we don't know what we don't know.

Introduction

This book aims to highlight an essential aspect of our clinical work: the clinician's attunement to the client.

The client has an outer presentation, which is essentially a response to day-to-day life: home, work, raising children, and having fun. Yet, in their inner world, they are feeling the effects of everything and anything that has ever happened to them. What is true—and we can see this by being more attuned to the client—is that a person's behavior, or lack thereof, is a direct reflection of how they have learned to cope with issues and events in their lives.

EMDR therapy, as described by Francine Shapiro, emphasizes the balance of thoughts and feelings. Our protocol is designed to teach us how to do it in a very, *very* specific manner. However, what the protocol doesn't actually address is the clinician's intuitive prowess and how to work with the client's timeline so that we are engaging with a neurological network, rather than simply treating each issue that arises in the client's life.

This is the basis for the art of attunement. It allows our clients to attach to their authentic selves—to the truths of their strength—through their therapeutic work with us.

The book is divided into several parts.

The first part discusses what attunement actually is and its effects on people.

EMDR can be incredibly effective for a wide range of people, but, like any approach, it's not a one-size-fits-all solution. EMDR processing might not be the best fit at certain times for clients who are in the middle of a severe crisis, actively using substances to the point that it interferes with processing, or who don't yet have the internal resources to stay grounded during emotional work. For example, individuals with untreated dissociative identity disorders

(DID) or unmanaged psychosis may need significant stabilization before engaging in trauma processing. That said, it's not necessarily that EMDR can't work for them; it just means we need to go at a different pace, with a strong focus on resourcing and stabilization first.

The beauty of EMDR is that it's adaptable. When we tailor the approach to the client's readiness and needs, even those who initially seem like they might not be a fit can benefit from the concept that frames the art of attunement. When the time is right, this is the thinking behind the art of attunement. We must consider the client's position and proceed with the EMDR protocol as it applies to the client, taking into account their ability and readiness. And if the client is not yet ready for the processing phase of EMDR therapy, we must take our time and attune to the client's needs.

Structure of the Book

This book is thoughtfully organized to provide a transparent and progressive journey through EMDR therapy. It begins with Section 1: **Foundations**, which explores the history, scientific principles, and theoretical frameworks underlying EMDR, establishing a strong conceptual base.

The second section, **Attunement in Therapy**, emphasizes the importance of attunement and its refined role within EMDR.

Moving into Section 3: **Practical Application**, the focus shifts to hands-on techniques, covering attunement within the eight phases of EMDR, resourcing strategies, and advanced methods.

The final section offers a concise synthesis of key insights and practical takeaways, equipping practitioners with actionable tools to enhance their therapeutic effectiveness.

The Importance of Balancing Theory and Practice in EMDR

A foundational aspect of this book is the recognition that effective therapeutic work rests on a harmonious integration of rigorous evidence-based theory and hands-on practice. It is only through the process of attunement to clients that a clinician can offer the best therapeutic experience. The art of attunement is a crucial yet challenging aspect in the process of forming a therapeutic alliance and achieving meaningful outcomes for the client.

While understanding the scientific underpinnings of EMDR provides clarity about its mechanisms and efficacy, it is equally crucial to appreciate the nuanced, real-world experiences that inform its application. The authors—Esta Porter and Cindi Saj—bring a rich mosaic of both scholarly knowledge and lived clinical expertise to this work, ensuring that the discussion remains grounded, relevant, and adaptable to diverse therapeutic contexts.

You will notice the first few chapters are grounded in research, while the later sections of the book are based on professional experience and practice. We aim to provide information grounded in evidence-based research and translate concepts that are applicable to clinical practice. We will achieve this by providing concrete illustrations that reflect real-world practices and techniques helpful in working with clients.

Combined, we have over 65 years of counseling experience. We have had the teachable moments, the clinical consultations, the case studies, and the learning journey that is worth sharing to make the field a better place.

Esta brings over 50 years of experience. She has taught at universities and assisted esteemed colleagues in editing their books. She has also contributed to research papers and completed many advanced EMDR trainings. The protocol detailed in this manuscript reflects how she works with clients. While she prefers not to conduct her own research—humorously stating, "I'd rather die than do so"—she relies on her extensive clinical experience, which is reflected in the eight-phase model outlined in this book.

As an EMDRIA-approved trainer, she presents EMDR in a way that draws from her work with thousands of clients and hundreds of consultations. Although the section may lack citations, it is deeply rooted in her practical knowledge and professional insights. Therefore, the absence of references is due to the nature of the material, which is primarily based on experiential expertise rather than formal academic sources.

The basic protocol is drawn—with great honor—from Francine Shapiro's lifelong work. Francine's commitment to making this world a better place is the cornerstone of Esta's intent. Each client or consultee she works with is seen as an individual being and has contributed to her ability to attune to the human experience and bring meaningful transitions to lives well-lived.

Dr. Cindi Saj has over 15 years of experience working with children, youth, and adults. She met Esta during an EMDR training, and Esta has been her mentor both within the field and beyond. Dr. Cindi is a dedicated Registered Social Worker and an EMDRIA-Certified EMDR Therapist. She is also an EMDRIA-Approved Consultant-in-Training.

By blending the authors' extensive life experiences, clinical practices, and deep understanding of EMDR's theoretical foundations, their insights and reflections serve as a bridge between the academic and experiential realms.

This book is a compilation of a learning journey into attunement and EMDR. The authors demonstrate how empirical research informs treatment strategies and how clinical insights can, in turn, refine and evolve theoretical models. This is a call to action (CTA) for increased awareness and reflection around the concept of attunement in EMDR.

Section 1
Foundations: History, Science, and Theory of EMDR

The Origins and Evolution of EMDR

In 1989, Francine Shapiro, a clinical therapist and researcher, was dealing with trauma related to her own health when she noticed something while walking in the woods. She found that moving her eyes back and forth provided her relief from her anxious feelings and thoughts. This discovery led her to explore the connection between eye movements and emotional state changes, ultimately resulting in the development of Eye Movement Desensitization and Reprocessing (EMDR) therapy.

After her initial findings, Shapiro continued to explore EMDR by studying 22 clients who had traumatic memories, such as those related to the Vietnam War and sexual abuse (Shapiro, 1989). She noticed that many of them struggled with issues like unwanted thoughts and difficulties in relationships. Many of these individuals faced challenges such as intrusive thoughts, flashbacks, trouble sleeping, low self-esteem, relationship problems, as well as anxiety, depression, and issues with substance abuse (Shapiro, 1989). Through her work with EMDR and trauma, she was able to help these individuals lessen the emotional pain tied to their traumatic memories (Shapiro, 1989; Shapiro, 1991).

As she helped them confront their painful experiences, their way of thinking began to change, leading them to develop more positive thoughts about themselves (Shapiro, 1991). The participants reported sleeping better, having fewer nightmares, and experiencing fewer flashbacks (Shapiro, 1991).

This body of research culminated in the creation of Eye Movement Desensitization and Reprocessing (EMDR) therapy, initially aimed at treating post-traumatic stress disorder (PTSD) in individuals affected by traumatic events. EMDR was proven effective in alleviating PTSD symptoms such as intrusive thoughts and flashbacks, as well as enhancing overall mental health and well-being (Shapiro, 1991).

Ever since it was first introduced, EMDR therapy has broadened its applications to tackle a diverse range of mental health concerns (Shapiro, 2001). It is now recognized for its effectiveness in treating conditions like anxiety, depression, PTSD, and other trauma-related issues. Notable organizations, including the American Psychological Association (APA), the World Health Organization (WHO), and the Department of Veterans Affairs (VA), have endorsed EMDR as a valid treatment option (Shapiro, 2017; WHO, 2013; VA, 2017).

Beyond PTSD, EMDR has also been utilized to help individuals cope with phobias, grief, eating disorders, and complicated relationships. Many clinicians and researchers have reported success in using EMDR to address childhood trauma, chronic pain issues linked to emotional distress, and even performance anxiety in athletes. This growing recognition reinforces EMDR's versatility and relevance in contemporary mental health treatment (Shapiro, 2018; Maxfield & Hyer, 2002).

How EMDR Works: Phases and the AIP Model

EMDR Therapy

Eye Movement Desensitization and Reprocessing (EMDR) therapy distinguishes itself among various psychological treatment modalities by uniquely acknowledging the significant impact of emotionally charged past experiences on an individual's present mental state. While many therapeutic approaches concentrate on addressing immediate concerns, EMDR places a strong emphasis on the deep-seated influence of prior traumas on emotional well-being, self-perception, and cognitive patterns. For example, a person may struggle with feelings of worthlessness even when they possess a rational understanding of their inherent value (Shapiro, 2018).

Central to EMDR therapy is the goal of dismantling these emotional barriers and helping individuals achieve a more balanced and adaptive emotional existence. The therapy incorporates rapid eye movements (or other forms of bilateral stimulation) to facilitate the reprocessing of traumatic memories, mimicking the brain's natural processes during sleep, which helps consolidate and integrate experiences (Van der Kolk, 2014). This innovative therapeutic technique promotes significant healing, as it allows individuals to revisit and reconstruct their trauma narratives within a supportive therapeutic context (Hofmann et al., 2012).

The activity of the brain during sleep serves as an insightful analogy for the functioning of EMDR therapy. During sleep, we progress through different stages, including non-REM (rapid eye movement) and REM phases, both of which play essential roles in processing distressing experiences and integrating them into our self-concept (Walker, 2017). EMDR replicates this natural rhythm by alternating guided eye movements with periods of reflection on present emotions. This dynamic interaction creates a space for individuals to reframe their memories, promoting a healthier, more positive outlook while alleviating longstanding emotional distress (Solomon & Rothbaum, 2004).

Initially developed by Francine Shapiro, EMDR therapy placed a strong emphasis on eye movements as the primary form of bilateral stimulation. EMDR employs a technique known as bilateral stimulation, which consists of sets of eye movements (20-24), during which clients focus on distressing incidents. This approach is designed to desensitize emotional responses to these memories and aims to "calm" the disturbances linked to traumatic experiences (Shapiro, 2001).

However, subsequent research has demonstrated that various types of bilateral stimulation—including auditory cues and tactile sensations—are equally effective in achieving therapeutic results. This technique, referred to as bilateral dual attention stimulus, helps to reduce the distress associated with traumatic memories, effectively disentangling these memories from their overwhelming emotions and cognitive patterns (Luber & Shapiro, 2003).

A key element in understanding EMDR's effectiveness lies in the relationship between trauma and neurological responses. EMDR focuses on the neurological networks that store memories of distress and trauma, highlighting the importance of understanding these connections within clients. These networks can be interrelated, meaning that addressing one traumatic experience may trigger thoughts and emotions associated with other related traumas (Van der Kolk, 2014). Traumatic experiences, whether emotional or physical, can forge debilitating associations between memories and feelings, often resulting in a "stuck" state characterized by increased arousal and lasting symptoms (Van der Kolk, 2014). EMDR therapy skillfully addresses these challenges; it not only assists individuals in confronting immediate issues but also facilitates the processing and release of past burdens, thereby fostering emotional resilience and personal growth (Hofmann et al., 2012).

Another critical aspect of understanding EMDR is the concept of *cognitive validity*. Cognitive validity involves establishing a subjective unit of disturbance, emphasizing the need to evaluate both negative beliefs arising from traumatic experiences and their corresponding positive affirmations. A Likert scale is employed to measure the subjective belief associated with these statements, which are rooted in core self-beliefs. In the context of the subjective unit of disturbance, a higher score indicates a greater level of disturbance. Conversely, for the validity of the cognition score, a high score reflects a strong belief in positive self-statements, while a low score suggests a diminished belief in one's positive attributes (Shapiro, 2001).

EMDR therapy stands out as a potent tool for healing, effectively tackling present emotional difficulties while revealing the profound effects of historical trauma. By leveraging the brain's inherent ability to process and adapt, EMDR facilitates emotional emancipation and personal reclamation, empowering individuals to transcend their past and pursue a more fulfilling and balanced life.

The Eight Phases of EMDR Therapy

- Phase 1: History and Treatment of EMDR Therapy
- Phase 2: Preparation
- Phase 3: Assessment
- Phase 4: Desensitization
- Phase 5: Installation
- Phase 6: Body Scan
- Phase 7: Closure
- Phase 8: Re-evaluation

EMDR therapy is a comprehensive, multi-phase method designed to promote healing from traumatic experiences. The process begins with a thorough evaluation, where the therapist reviews the client's history to identify specific triggers and significant traumatic events that may continue to exert an influence on their well-being (Shapiro, 2018). Following this assessment, the client enters the preparation phase, during which they learn self-regulation techniques and self-care strategies to manage their emotional responses effectively (Leeds, 2016).

The subsequent phases concentrate on the targeted reprocessing of traumatic memories. In the desensitization phase, the therapist utilizes EMDR techniques to disrupt the association between the traumatic memories and their triggers (Shapiro, 2001). This is followed by the installation phase, in which the therapist assists the client in replacing negative thoughts with positive, empowering beliefs (Hofmann et al., 2012).

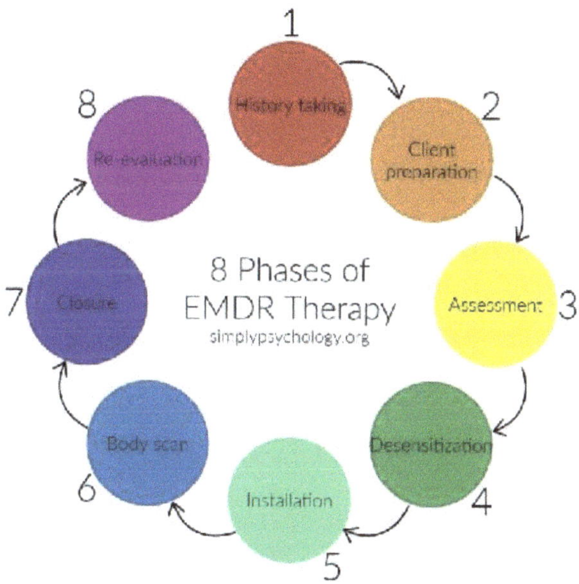

The body scan phase aims to address any residual physical symptoms associated with the trauma, ensuring that these manifestations are also processed (Shapiro, 2001). In the closure phase, the therapist plays a crucial role in helping the client return to a state of emotional equilibrium through the use of relaxation techniques (Hofmann et al., 2012).

Finally, in the re-evaluation phase, the therapist assesses the effectiveness of the treatment and determines whether the client's distress levels have decreased, ensuring that progress has been made in the therapeutic journey (Shapiro, 2018).

EMDR is grounded in research that validates its effectiveness in treating trauma and PTSD, supported by various clinical trials and meta-analyses (e.g., Cuijpers et al., 2016; Shapiro, 2018; Hase et al., 2019). The structured phases of EMDR therapy—preparation, assessment, desensitization, installation, body scan, closure, and re-evaluation—offer a scientific framework for trauma treatment (Shapiro, 2001).

However, the true skill in EMDR lies in the therapist's capacity to adapt the methodology to meet the individualized needs of each client, including the negotiation of bilateral stimulation techniques and the management of emotional reactions during processing. This combination of evidence-based protocols and personalized creativity enables therapists to build deeper connections with clients, thereby enriching the therapeutic experience (Leeds, 2016).

In this manner, EMDR is often considered both an art and a science due to its integration of structured therapeutic techniques with the clinician's intuitive and creative abilities (Shapiro, 2018). We will explore EMDR as both a science and an art in more detail next.

The Science Behind EMDR

EMDR Is Evidence-Based

EMDR is grounded in several psychological theories, notably the Adaptive Information Processing (AIP) model, which asserts that trauma can interfere with the brain's ability to process information effectively. This model posits that EMDR aids clients in reprocessing traumatic memories, promoting adaptive resolution and integration of these experiences (Shapiro, 2018).

EMDR is backed by an expanding array of scientific evidence, encompassing meta-analyses, randomized controlled trials, and neuroscientific studies (Watts et al., 2013). Its recognition as an effective treatment for PTSD and various trauma-related conditions underscores its scientific validity, as well as the need for continued research to understand its mechanisms and potential applications.

Furthermore, recent investigations using neuroimaging techniques have revealed alterations in brain activity associated with trauma processing both during and after EMDR treatment, supporting its neurobiological underpinnings (Hogberg et al., 2020).

Research Studies of EMDR

Multiple meta-analyses have validated the effectiveness of EMDR in treating PTSD. Research by Lee and Cuijpers (2013), Lee et al. (2016), and Papageorgiou et al. (2020) reviewed a range of studies and found that EMDR significantly alleviates PTSD symptoms in both children and adults when compared to control groups. Additionally, a comprehensive meta-analysis by Hill et al. (2020) confirmed EMDR's effectiveness for PTSD, showing that it leads to substantial reductions in symptoms compared to control conditions.

Francine Shapiro's original studies from 1989 demonstrated the efficacy of EMDR for PTSD treatment. In randomized controlled trials, participants exhibited significant decreases in PTSD symptoms after just a few sessions, with many experiencing complete relief from trauma-related distress. Further research by Van der Kolk et al. (2007), published in the *Journal of Traumatic Stress*, compared EMDR to other PTSD therapies, revealing that EMDR was as effective as cognitive behavioral therapy (CBT) and offered faster symptom relief, making it a compelling option for trauma treatment.

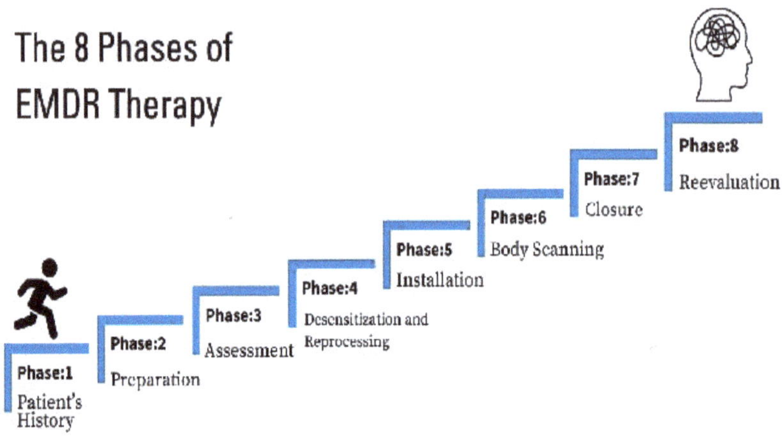

A meta-analysis by Hofmann et al. (2012) supported these findings, reviewing numerous studies on various psychotherapies for anxiety disorders and concluding that EMDR demonstrated strong efficacy in reducing anxiety and trauma symptoms, underscoring its status as an evidence-based treatment.

EMDR and Cultural Considerations

Cultural considerations are crucial when implementing EMDR therapy, as the process of attunement can vary markedly across different cultural backgrounds (Harris & Caspi, 2010). Harris and Caspi emphasize that cultural factors significantly shape both the therapeutic process and outcomes in EMDR, underscoring the importance of therapists demonstrating cultural sensitivity and attunement. Recognizing that cultural norms influence how clients perceive trauma, express emotions, and engage with therapy is vital for effective treatment (Shapiro, 2018). This understanding ensures that EMDR interventions are adapted to meet the unique cultural needs of each individual, thereby fostering greater engagement and more positive results.

For instance, children from diverse cultural contexts may interpret and respond to EMDR differently, necessitating approaches that respect their cultural schemas and communication styles (Hodge & Nadir, 2018). Similarly, clients from non-Western backgrounds might hold distinct beliefs about mental health and healing practices, requiring therapists to modify techniques to ensure cultural relevance and sensitivity (Kira et al., 2014). Brown (2013) emphasizes that cultural competence is essential in trauma therapy, advocating for clinicians to develop awareness, sensitivity, and adaptable strategies to serve diverse populations effectively. In the context of EMDR, such tailored approaches can strengthen the therapeutic alliance, promote safety, and optimize trauma processing within clients' cultural frameworks.

Cultural Sensitivity in EMDR Practice

Spear Chief (2017) has long emphasized the importance of integrating cultural awareness into therapeutic practice, noting that such integration fosters trust, safety, and active engagement in therapy. She asserts that this approach ultimately enhances treatment effectiveness, especially for Indigenous and marginalized communities (Spear Chief 2017).

In their research on the cross-cultural application of EMDR, Paulson and Spear Chief (2019) underscore the critical importance of integrating cultural awareness into therapy to ensure culturally sensitive treatment. They advocate for clinicians to have a deep understanding of clients' cultural backgrounds, as this enhances therapeutic rapport and improves treatment efficacy (Paulson & Spear Chief, 2019).

In a subsequent study, Paulson and Spear Chief (2020) examine the challenges and barriers to implementing EMDR across diverse cultural contexts. They identify key obstacles such as language differences, cultural stigma surrounding mental health, and varying expressions of trauma and trauma narratives. These findings underscore the importance of clinicians being culturally attuned, competent, and adaptable in their approach. The researchers also emphasize the importance of developing culturally adapted EMDR protocols to better align with specific cultural contexts, thereby fostering more effective and respectful therapeutic interventions (Paulson & Spear Chief, 2020).

Paulson and Spear Chief (2022) also conducted research comparing standard EMDR approaches with culturally adapted versions. The findings demonstrated the benefits of tailoring interventions to clients' cultural backgrounds and revealed that integrating cultural considerations into EMDR enhances client engagement, leading to a greater reduction in symptoms (Paulson & Spear Chief, 2022).

As a result, integrating cultural considerations into EMDR therapy is essential for maximizing its effectiveness across diverse populations. Recognizing and respecting clients' cultural backgrounds not only strengthens the therapeutic alliance but also facilitates more meaningful engagement and successful trauma processing. As research by Harris and Caspi (2010), Spear Chief (2017), and Paulson and Spear Chief (2019, 2020, 2022) illustrates, culturally adapted approaches lead to better outcomes, particularly for Indigenous and marginalized communities.

Therefore, clinicians are encouraged to develop cultural competence and incorporate culturally sensitive modifications into their EMDR practices, ensuring that therapy is both respectful and effective in addressing the unique needs of their clients.

Neurobiology of Attunement and SPECT Scan Insights

Emerging neuroimaging research has greatly enhanced our understanding of how therapeutic interventions influence brain function, with recent studies specifically highlighting the neural effects of EMDR therapy. One such technique, Single Photon Emission

Computed Tomography (SPECT) scans, utilizes small amounts of radioactive material to visualize and measure brain activity and function. In the context of PTSD and EMDR, SPECT scans have offered valuable insights into the changes occurring within the brain's structure and activity in individuals undergoing treatment. These findings contribute to a growing body of evidence supporting the neurobiological basis of EMDR's effectiveness (Luber & Lisanby, 2014).

For example, a case study of a war veteran with severe PTSD who underwent EMDR treatment revealed notable brain changes. Before therapy, SPECT scans revealed heightened activity in the amygdala, linked to fear and emotional reactivity, and reduced activity in the prefrontal cortex, which is involved in regulation and decision-making. After completing EMDR sessions, follow-up scans demonstrated decreased amygdala activity, indicating less emotional reactivity, and increased activity in the prefrontal cortex, suggesting improved emotional regulation. Clinically, the veteran reported a significant reduction in flashbacks and anxiety, illustrating how neural changes align with symptom improvement (Fateh et al., 2017).

Studies have shown considerable alterations in brain activity and function following EMDR therapy. Notably, SPECT scans indicate that EMDR can lead to a reduction in amygdala activity, suggesting diminished emotional reactivity (Pagani et al., 2018). Moreover, EMDR therapy has been associated with increased activity in the prefrontal cortex, which may contribute to enhanced emotional regulation and improved decision-making skills. SPECT scans have also indicated reduced glucose metabolism in the brain following EMDR, which may imply a decrease in emotional arousal and reactivity (Fateh et al., 2017). Additionally, the therapy appears to enhance blood flow to the prefrontal cortex, which may correlate with improved executive functioning and emotional regulation (Baek et al., 2018). These observations offer profound insights into the neural mechanisms that support EMDR's efficacy in addressing PTSD and other trauma-related conditions (Müller et al., 2018; Lee & Cuijpers, 2013).

Research has shown that EMDR therapy can lead to significant changes in brain activity and function, which are associated with reduced symptoms of PTSD and other trauma-related disorders. Studies have demonstrated that EMDR therapy can reduce amygdala activity, indicating a decrease in emotional reactivity (Lanius et al., 2010). Additionally, the therapy has been found to increase activity in the prefrontal cortex, which may be related to improved emotional regulation and decision-making (Kim et al., 2011). Furthermore, EMDR therapy has been linked to decreased glucose metabolism in the brain, potentially indicating a reduction in emotional arousal and reactivity (Goldsmith et al., 2014). The therapy has also been shown to increase blood flow to the prefrontal cortex, which may be related to improved executive function and emotional regulation (Ludascher et al., 2012). Moreover, EMDR therapy has been found to alter activity in the default mode network, which is involved in self-referential processing and memory consolidation (Bremner et al., 2012).

These findings collectively suggest that EMDR therapy may lead to changes in brain activity and function that are associated with reduced symptoms of PTSD and other trauma-related disorders.

These studies suggest that EMDR therapy may result in alterations in brain activity and function that correlate with a reduction in symptoms of PTSD and other trauma-related disorders (Hofmann et al., 2012). For instance, in a clinical case series, a patient with chronic PTSD showed marked symptom improvement after EMDR treatment, accompanied by decreased activity in fear-related brain regions and increased activity in areas associated with emotional regulation, as measured by SPECT scans (Shapiro, 2014).

SPECT imaging has provided insights into the neurological changes experienced by individuals with PTSD, particularly those undergoing EMDR therapy. Research suggests that EMDR may induce changes in brain activity and function, potentially leading to enhanced emotional regulation, reduced emotional reactivity, and improved executive functioning. These results support the efficacy of EMDR as a therapeutic modality for addressing PTSD and related trauma disorders. However, it is crucial to acknowledge that these findings are derived from individual studies and might not represent the experiences of all patients with PTSD or those receiving EMDR. Additional research is needed to fully understand the neural mechanisms that underpin EMDR's effectiveness in treating PTSD and to broaden its therapeutic applications (Shapiro, 2014).

In summary, neuroimaging studies—particularly those utilizing SPECT—offer compelling evidence that EMDR therapy induces meaningful neurobiological changes, such as reduced amygdala activity, increased prefrontal engagement, and alterations in brain networks, that correlate with clinical improvements in PTSD symptoms. These insights reinforce EMDR's role as a potent trauma-focused intervention and underscore the importance of ongoing research to elucidate its neural underpinnings, ultimately guiding more targeted and effective treatments for trauma-related disorders.

Section 2
Attunement in Therapy:
The Therapist-Client Relationship

Defining Attunement and Its Clinical Significance

What Is Attunement?

Attunement refers to the capacity to recognize, comprehend, and respond appropriately to another individual's emotional state and needs (Siegel, 2010). It can be described as a kinesthetic and emotional ability to sense and connect with others, understanding their rhythm, feelings, and experiences as if being in their skin (Stern, 1985; Foscha, 2000).

Attunement goes beyond mere empathy. It creates a reciprocal, resonant experience of shared feeling and unbroken connectedness between individuals. This deep form of emotional connection fosters genuine understanding and emotional safety, both of which are essential for meaningful relationships and personal growth (Stern, 1985).

From birth, humans are wired for attunement. Even before conception, through the processes of ovulation and fertilization, innate attunement guides our biological and emotional development (Schore, 2003). The fetus remains attuned to the environment of the womb—responding to warmth, comfort, and stimuli—demonstrating that attunement is an inherent feature of our existence. As we grow, this primal capacity continues to develop, forming the foundation for our ability to connect, understand, and navigate the world (Schore, 2003).

Attunement is similar to, yet distinct from, empathy and therapeutic alliance (Ogden & Fisher, 2015). It requires a conscious and nuanced awareness of another person's emotional state, along with the ability to respond appropriately to their needs in the moment. Unlike empathy, which involves understanding and sharing the feelings of another (Brown, 2010), attunement emphasizes presence and receptivity to subtle cues, facilitating deep connection and trust (Siegel, 2010). Note the chart describing the definition, purpose, and anticipated outcome of the process of attunement, therapeutic alliance, and empathy:

Process	Attunement (Siegel, 2010)	**Therapeutic Alliance** (Nienhuis et al., 2018)	Empathy (Brown, 2010)
Definiton	The ability to tune into and understand another person's emotional state in the moment	A collaborative and trusting relationship between individuals or groups working toward common goals	The capacity to understand and share the feelings of another person
Purpose	To connect deeply on an emotional level and respond appropriately.	To build a strong, effective working or relational bond.	To understand and validate another's emotional experience.
Outcome	Enhanced emotional connection and understanding.	Increased trust, cooperation, and shared commitment.	Greater compassion, trust, and emotional rapport.

A therapeutic alliance, by contrast, refers to a collaborative and goal-oriented relationship characterized by mutual commitment and shared purpose (Nienhuis et al., 2018). Empathy is the capacity to understand and share the feelings of another person (Brown, 2010). Attunement serves as the foundational relational skill that enhances empathy and supports the development of a strong alliance by ensuring that interactions are sensitive, responsive, and aligned with the individual's emotional experiences (Siegel, 2010).

A lack of attunement, either with oneself or others, is often at the root of feelings of dissatisfaction, dysfunction, and unhappiness. When individuals are disconnected from their own internal experiences or from those around them, it can hinder their ability to live in a happy, adaptive, and successful manner (Schore, 2003). Recognizing this, therapeutic practices emphasize helping clients develop greater attunement to their inner worlds, to others, and to the often-hidden aspects of themselves.

In therapy, fostering attunement involves creating a safe space where clients can explore aspects of themselves that they may wish to avoid or are not yet aware of. A therapist's nonjudgmental acceptance and attuned presence reassure clients that they are understood and safe to be their authentic selves. This environment encourages clients to become more conscious of their defenses and inner experiences, paving the way for meaningful change and personal growth.

Ultimately, attunement is a fundamental and innate aspect of being human—an intrinsic part of how we understand and relate to the universe and ourselves (Sweeney & Myers, 2023). It is the foundation upon which all meaningful connections and healing are built. With this understanding, we can better appreciate the role of attunement in therapeutic practices, including EMDR therapy, as well as the art of fostering genuine human connection (Sweeney & Myers, 2023).

During the counseling process, numerous key factors must be considered to ensure effective outcomes (McLeod, 2015). Among these considerations is the importance of a counselor establishing a strong therapeutic alliance with the client (Norcross & Lambert, 2018). To connect with the client, a counselor must communicate that the client is in a safe and supportive environment and that they are valued and understood (Sweeney & Myers, 2023). The client must, in turn, believe that the counselor is a trustworthy resource, enabling them to feel safe and secure enough to participate fully in the therapeutic process.

A counselor is trained to engage in active listening, demonstrate empathy, and maintain a nonjudgmental attitude. These expectations are crucial in fostering trust and confidence. Research suggests that trust from the client toward the counselor significantly enhances the effectiveness of the counseling process (Meyer & Turner, 2023). It is also essential for counselors to utilize personalized therapeutic approaches tailored to each client's unique experiences and emotional landscape, as this fosters more meaningful healing (Kivlighan & Tully, 2023).

Additionally, expanding knowledge of counseling theory beyond the basics is crucial. Although foundational training in counseling is important, gaining a deeper and more nuanced understanding and application can greatly enhance therapeutic outcomes (Watkins & Riggs, 2023).

Furthermore, in the world of counseling, the therapist's intuition plays a significant role. Therapists need to cultivate and trust their intuition to connect with clients and support them in their healing processes (Miller & Rollnick, 2023).

The significance of attunement in therapy lies in its ability to align with the client's needs and emotional state, ultimately enhancing therapeutic effectiveness and yielding more favorable outcomes (Siegel, 2010).

Building the Therapeutic Alliance Through Presence

Attunement in the Therapeutic Framework

Within a therapeutic framework, attunement reflects the counselor's ability and skill in forming an emotional connection with the client, characterized by empathy, sensitivity, and validation of their experiences (Siegel, 2010). When a counselor attunes to their client, they are actively tuning in to and engaging with the client's emotional and psychological experience. By establishing this emotional bond, attunement fosters a sense of safety and trust, allowing clients to engage more deeply and effectively in the therapeutic process. This emotional synchrony is crucial for facilitating meaningful change and healing in therapy (Ogden & Minton, 2000).

Siegel (2010) emphasizes the importance of attunement in the therapeutic relationship, defining it as the therapist's ability to respond sensitively to a client's emotional needs. He argues that attunement fosters safety and trust, which are essential for deeper understanding and healing. Additionally, he suggests that mindfulness and neural integration enhance a therapist's capacity to attune, resulting in improved client engagement and therapeutic outcomes.

Similarly, Hase, Goldstein, and Schmid (2016) discuss the significance of attunement in EMDR therapy, highlighting that the therapist's connection with the client's emotional state is crucial for effective treatment. They point out that a responsive and empathetic therapeutic alliance facilitates the reprocessing of traumatic memories and provides practical strategies for achieving attunement, such as nonverbal communication and active listening. Their holistic approach emphasizes the integration of EMDR techniques with interpersonal dynamics, suggesting that strong attunement leads to improved therapeutic outcomes and greater client satisfaction.

In summary, both studies emphasize that attunement is crucial for creating a safe therapeutic environment, facilitating deeper healing through effective engagement with the client's emotional experiences. This underscores the critical role of the therapeutic relationship in successful trauma treatment.

Attunement in therapy is a foundational aspect that speaks to the therapist's ability to be emotionally aware and responsive to their client's needs (Siegel, 2010). Effective attunement in the therapeutic relationship involves not only a verbal understanding of the client's communication but also a profound sensitivity to their emotional nuances and nonverbal expressions. This includes being attuned to subtle cues such as body language, facial expressions, and tone of voice, as well as an empathetic understanding of their underlying emotions and experiences (Siegel, 2010; Hase, Goldstein, & Schmid, 2016).

This sensitivity is particularly crucial in EMDR therapy, which involves processing traumatic memories and emotions that often arise during the treatment (Shapiro, 2014). In EMDR, the therapist's role is to observe the client's reactions throughout various treatment phases closely. This vigilant observation helps identify emotional shifts, such as signs of distress, comfort, or readiness to move on to the next phase. By being attuned to these signals, the therapist can adjust their approach in real-time, ensuring that the treatment remains aligned with the client's emotional state (Hase et al., 2016). This responsiveness enhances the therapeutic alliance and creates a safe space for the client to explore and process their traumatic experiences more effectively (Norcross, 2011).

Attunement is particularly crucial in the initial stages of therapy, where establishing rapport and trust is vital. During this phase, the therapist's ability to connect with the client can significantly influence the effectiveness of the therapeutic process. Clients are more likely to engage openly and share their experiences if they feel understood and supported (Safran & Muran, 2000).

In EMDR, the resourcing stage is particularly important for attunement, as it involves creating a foundation of safety and stability. During this stage, the therapist works with the client to identify personal strengths, coping strategies, and positive memories that can serve as emotional anchors throughout the trauma processing. The connection forged between the client and counselor during this phase is vital, as it not only nurtures trust but also equips the client with internal resources to manage the emotional challenges that may arise during subsequent stages of EMDR (Shapiro, 2014).

Attunement and the Therapeutic Process

Overall, attunement is a dynamic and ongoing process that enhances the effectiveness of therapy. It allows the therapist to respond adaptively to the client's needs, promoting emotional healing and resilience in the face of trauma. By cultivating a strong therapeutic relationship grounded in empathy and understanding, the therapist can facilitate deeper processing and transformation for the client (Perry, 2009).

Attunement in Resourcing and Stabilization

EMDR: Attunement and Resourcing

Within counseling, attunement begins the moment the counselor and client meet and continues throughout the EMDR process. When clients first arrive for therapy, they may still be uncertain about whether they can trust the therapist with their struggles. This is where attunement becomes vital. In EMDR therapy, while we follow a structured protocol, it becomes clear with experience that attentively responding to the client's unique needs within that framework is paramount.

Attunement is crucial for the therapist to be in tune with their clients, as it enhances the efficacy of therapy by fostering a deeper understanding of the client's emotional and psychological state (Norcross, 2011). This connection enables the clinician to tailor interventions more effectively. Likewise, it is equally important for the client to attune to their therapist. This mutual attunement fosters trust and safety, which are essential components of therapeutic engagement. When clients feel understood and supported, they are more likely to engage fully in the process, facilitating significant emotional processing and healing (Shapiro, 2018).

This concept has been supported by research, emphasizing the importance of the therapeutic alliance and the emotional connection between therapist and client in promoting positive outcomes in psychotherapy (Norcross, 2011). The attunement between a counselor and client is not only vital for creating trust but also for establishing a safe space where the client can explore their emotions and feelings. Research indicates that a strong therapeutic alliance significantly enhances the healing process (Norcross & Lambert, 2018).

Attunement is especially crucial in the resourcing process, as it ensures that clients are in a favorable mental state that promotes healing. Before entering the EMDR processing phase, clients must feel grounded and supported. This emotional stability enables them to fully engage in the therapeutic work, thereby improving the overall efficacy of the EMDR technique. In this way, establishing strong attunement serves as a precursor to effective resourcing, ultimately leading to more profound healing experiences (Levy & Orlans, 2016).

Looking Ahead: The Role of Resourcing in Therapy

In the upcoming sections of this book, we will explore how clinicians can effectively assist clients during the resourcing process. This stage serves several key purposes, primarily to stabilize the client at the outset of treatment and alleviate feelings of overwhelm, dissociation, distress, or discomfort. Clients are encouraged to utilize these resources before, during, and after sessions to self-soothe.

The therapist must remain attuned during this stage, allowing them to connect deeply with the client and "read the room"—gauging the client's level of engagement and emotional presence. This attunement, paired with effective resourcing techniques, supports both therapist and client in being present, attentive, and emotionally available for the therapeutic work ahead. Proper preparation through resourcing significantly improves therapy outcomes by ensuring the client is mentally and emotionally ready for reprocessing.

Understanding which resourcing strategies to employ is vital, as not all clients will respond to the same techniques. Building a strong rapport is essential in helping clients identify and use tools that genuinely resonate with them. During the exploration of resources and the psychoeducation phase, we will emphasize the importance of intuitive clinical judgment and the necessity of customizing approaches to suit each client's individual needs.

Therapist and Client Attunement

Throughout the entire therapeutic journey, attunement allows the therapist to remain sensitive to the client's emotional state, fostering an atmosphere of safety and validation that is essential for healing (Leeds, 2016). By being responsive to the client's needs, emotions, and experiences, the therapist creates an environment that fosters the development of positive attributes, such as self-awareness, self-acceptance, self-compassion, and inner peace.

Attunement is a vital component of the EMDR therapeutic process, as it facilitates a strong connection between the therapist and the client. When therapists are attuned, they foster an environment of trust and safety, enabling clients to feel heard, understood, and validated in their experiences (Shapiro, 2018).

Conversely, when clients experience attunement from their therapist, they are more likely to have confidence in the therapeutic process.

This mutual attunement enhances the ability of both the client and the therapist to process the client's emotions effectively, which is essential for reprocessing traumatic memories and facilitating emotional healing (Leeds, 2016). By maintaining attunement, the therapist can amplify empathy, minimize countertransference, and increase self-awareness—all of which contribute to a more effective and efficient therapeutic experience (Hofmann et al., 2012).

Moreover, attunement plays a significant role in promoting long-term recovery by cultivating a sense of safety, trust, and connection within the therapeutic relationship. This foundational aspect ultimately supports the client's emotional healing and personal growth, making it essential for the success of the therapeutic journey (Siegel, 2010).

The Eight Phases

Resourcing and Advanced Techniques

Understanding the Role of Attunement

Throughout the eight phases of EMDR therapy, attunement is crucial for fostering a therapeutic relationship founded on trust, empathy, and understanding. Beginning with Phase 1, where the therapist establishes a safe and welcoming environment for clients to share their experiences, and continuing through Phase 8, which involves helping clients process any lingering emotions or thoughts, attunement is essential for nurturing a sense of connection and mutual comprehension (Shapiro, 2018).

During the assessment phase (Phase 3), the therapist evaluates the client's distress levels and their capacity for processing (Phase 4), demonstrating flexibility and adaptability by adjusting the treatment plan to suit the client's unique needs. In the desensitization phase (Phase 5), the therapist uses bilateral stimulation to support the processing and integration of traumatic memories, fostering a sense of calm and resolution (Hofmann et al., 2012).

When individuals seek counseling, they bring with them a deeply ingrained cognitive and emotional framework shaped by their life experiences and interactions with the world. The cumulative effect of these experiences, including trauma, triggers specific responses that initially serve as adaptive and protective mechanisms. However, over time, these responses may become limiting and maladaptive, reinforced by the brain due to their previous effectiveness.

During the initial preparation stage, the goal is to help the client access a more resilient and adaptive neurological network. This process enables them to process better and manage trauma, equipping them with tools and strategies to handle future challenges. By guiding the client through this foundational phase, we create a supportive environment in which they can safely explore and work through past experiences.

In standard EMDR protocols, preparation begins before the start of the reprocessing phase of EMDR therapy and involves creating a sense of security for the client. This is achieved by providing an environment, both physically and psychologically, that promotes calm and safety. The preparation phase begins during the rapport-building process, even before the formal intake process. It is designed to ensure the client is emotionally prepared and capable of being present during the processing, reprocessing, and stabilization stages. The preparation phase encompasses various techniques designed to enhance the client's emotional resilience and lay a solid foundation for the therapeutic work ahead.

A vital component of this phase is helping clients develop grounding and containment strategies. These techniques enable clients to manage overwhelming feelings and avoid dissociation or resistance that could hinder the healing process.

Resourcing Techniques for EMDR

Incorporating resourcing techniques is essential across counseling approaches to foster feelings of safety, security, and comfort. Often referred to as coping strategies or skills, resourcing encompasses a wide range of physical, psychological, and cognitive methods (Hensley, 2020). For example, grounding techniques help clients stay mindful and present in the moment while breathing exercises support calmness. Cognitive tools such as counting or distraction methods empower individuals to handle triggering situations with greater ease and composure.

Within the context of EMDR therapy, resourcing plays a crucial role in helping individuals cultivate a sense of calm, safety, comfort, and bodily connection, which is especially important when processing traumatic memories (Hensley, 2020).

During the resourcing phase, the therapist introduces various techniques to help the client feel more grounded and connected to their body, emotions, and thoughts. The primary goal is to foster calm and safety, reducing anxiety, disconnection, and hyperarousal. These approaches help individuals become more present and anchored in their bodies, reduce fear and anxiety, encourage a sense of peace, and allow for more efficient and effective trauma processing.

Check-in

In the process of self-reflection and healing, it is crucial to establish a foundation of self-awareness and engage in regular self-check-ins. This practice enables individuals to monitor their emotional state and identify areas that require attention and improvement. It involves acknowledging and accepting one's emotions, thoughts, and physical sensations in the present moment, without judgment or attachment.

Within EMDR, this process is typically initiated at the beginning of a session, serving as a means for both the therapist and the client to assess the client's current level of awareness and capacity for self-reflection. Through a self-check-in, important information can emerge, such as whether the client is dissociating and needs grounding or resourcing at the moment.

To conduct a check-in, the therapist may ask the client to rate their current level of comfort on a scale of 1 to 5, where 1 indicates extreme discomfort and 5 indicates extreme comfort. If the client reports feeling at a 1 or say 2, the therapist can then draw upon specific resources to help stabilize and secure the therapeutic space.

Ideas for a Check-In

Here's an example of how a therapist might guide a client through this process:

"Take a moment to notice how you're feeling right now. On a scale of 1 to 5, where 5 is extremely comfortable and 1 is extremely uncomfortable, how would you rate your current level of comfort?"

Clients can then share their comfort level, which not only supports attunement but also helps assess dissociation and overall readiness for the session.

After determining the client's level of comfort and readiness, the next step involves identifying a presenting issue and examining the associated thoughts, feelings, and physical sensations. This provides valuable insight into the client's current internal state, allowing the therapist to tailor the session's approach accordingly. During this process, the therapist might ask:

- *"How are you feeling emotionally?"*
- *"What are you noticing right now?"*
- *"Are you experiencing any physical sensations or tension?"*
- *"Is there anything causing you discomfort or distress?"*

Jim Knipe, in his book EMDR Toolbox, refers to this check-in as securing the space. If there is any discomfort, it's wise to ask what would make this better. And how comfortable does the client feel in this space? Also, ask how comfortable the client feels being with you, the clinician. In addition, we ask how we can ensure that we are feeling secure enough both in the space and with us as a clinician, so that this information registers within the client's system.

Takeaway

By conducting regular check-ins before beginning a counseling session, and especially in EMDR, therapists and clients can better connect to the emotional tone of the moment and assess readiness and comfort levels. It is also an effective way for therapists to gauge their attunement to the client by eliminating the need to guess. Honest, collaborative check-ins establish the groundwork for a strong therapeutic alliance. Moreover, they help clients identify and name their thoughts and feelings, which enhances self-awareness.

The check-in is a key part of the preparation phase in EMDR and should not be overlooked.

Emotional Awareness

Like the check-in, being aware of and in tune with one's emotions in the present moment is essential. Some individuals naturally possess strong emotional awareness, while others may struggle to recognize and name their feelings.

Emotional awareness is critical on the path to healing. The key to working effectively with emotions lies in the ability to identify and differentiate them. Emotions range from anger, disgust, sadness, and surprise to happiness, excitement, and many others. Once an individual can accurately identify a feeling, they can begin to understand it and explore its roots.

Research on EMDR and core beliefs suggests that the strength of an individual's emotional response to triggering events is closely tied to the age at which an emotional disturbance first appeared (Shapiro, 2001). Specifically, studies have shown that the earlier the disturbance occurred, the more intense the emotional response is likely to be. This underscores the importance of addressing early life experiences and traumatic events when working to heal emotional distress.

When individuals become aware of a disturbance or traumatic event, they often form a deeply rooted belief about themselves that is intricately linked to their sense of identity (Young et al., 2003). This belief, whether true or false, can significantly affect their self-concept and worldview. The repetition of distressing events reinforces the belief, making it more resistant to change over time. If the emotional distress becomes overwhelming, individuals may adopt coping strategies such as avoidance, emotional shutdown, or dissociation to shield themselves from further psychological pain.

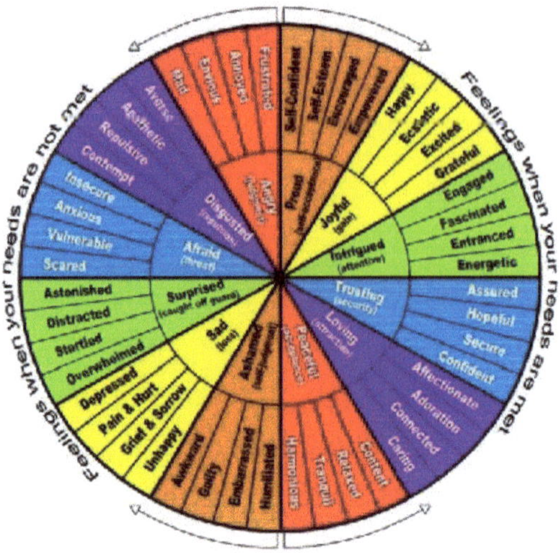

Developing emotional literacy, which involves having both the language and awareness of one's emotions, is essential for effective self-regulation and resourcing. It enables individuals to understand their emotional experiences more effectively, process them more efficiently, and manage them more effectively (Gross & John, 2003). This Emotions Wheel helps us recognize and increase awareness of our feelings. It also helps identify the emotions that emerge when our needs are fulfilled, as well as name those feelings that appear when our needs are unmet.

- How to Instruct and Encourage Emotional Awareness
- Create a Safe Environment
- Use Mindfulness Techniques to reflect on emotions
- Allow Space to Unpack and Discuss Emotions
- Practice Regular Check-Ins

Takeaway

Encouraging emotional awareness is an ongoing journey that requires both patience and consistent practice. By creating a safe enough space, using mindfulness tools, and incorporating regular check-ins, individuals become more in tune with their emotions. This awareness fosters deeper interpersonal connections and strengthens emotional intelligence over time. The key lies in the clinician being steady, supportive, and receptive to the evolving landscape of emotional understanding.

Being aware of and in sync with one's emotional experience is foundational to the healing process. Emotional awareness refers to recognizing and understanding one's feelings, which can then be further explored and measured using techniques such as scaling. However, if the emotional underlay is acquired before language and cognitive understanding are available to the client, then the felt sense of the emotions may be understood as a bodily sensation.

Scaling

Scaling in counseling is a technique used to help clients quantify and visualize their feelings, thoughts, or behaviors (De Jong & Berg, 2013). It involves asking clients to rate their experience on a numerical scale, typically ranging from 1 to 10, where 1 represents the lowest or most difficult feeling, and 10 describes the highest or most positive feeling state. For example, a scale from 1 to 10 can be used to measure levels of happiness, disturbance, anxiety, motivation, or safety.

The primary purposes of scaling are to improve communication, increase self-awareness, and track client progress. Scaling makes feelings and behaviors measurable, enabling both clients and therapists to assess the intensity, frequency, and improvement over time. For example, when used behaviorally, a scale may reflect how often a behavior occurs, 1 meaning "almost never" and 10 meaning "all the time."

In EMDR therapy, the most commonly used scale is the Subjective Units of Disturbance (SUD) scale, which helps determine the emotional intensity. The primary aim of EMDR is often to reduce emotional reactivity, so having a consistent way to measure and reflect on distress is critical.

The SUD scale enables both the therapist and the client to quantify the level of emotional disturbance associated with a specific thought, memory, or situation. It plays an integral role before, during, and after trauma processing. Being able to name and measure emotional responses contributes significantly to self-awareness and emotional regulation. The scale also enhances communication, creating a shared language that helps clients articulate their emotional states while enabling therapists to adjust their interventions accordingly.

Instructions for Scaling with SUD

1. ***Identify the Situation***

   Reflect on the current situation, event, or thought that is causing distress. This could be a specific memory, an ongoing concern, or a general sense of unease.

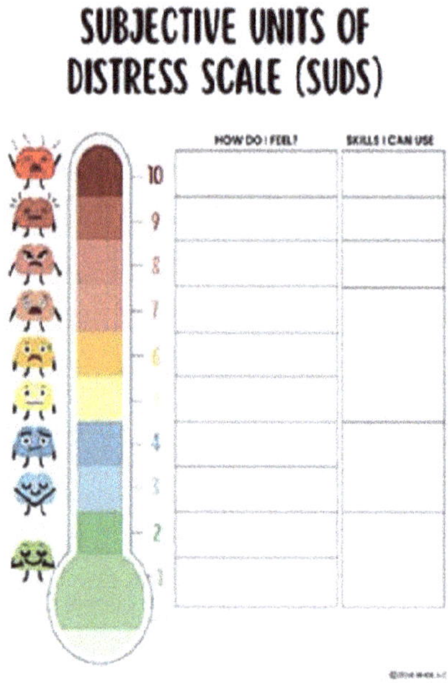

2. ***Subjective Units of Disturbance Scaling***

   1: No distress (calm, neutral feelings)

   1–3: Mild distress (slightly uncomfortable, manageable)

   4–6: Moderate distress (noticeable impact, somewhat overwhelming)

   7–9: Severe distress (intense discomfort, significant functional impact)

   10: Extreme distress (panic, crisis-level discomfort)

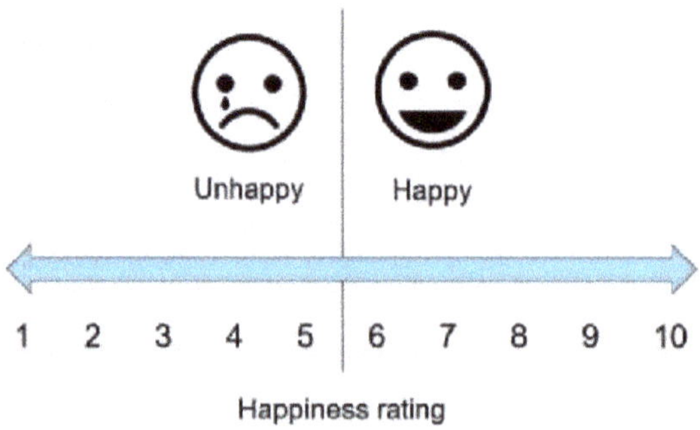

Apply the Scale

Ask the client to choose the number that best represents their current level of distress.

The SUD scale can be used at various points during EMDR treatment, including at the start of a session, during desensitization, and at the end of processing. It helps indicate the degree of disturbance initially felt and tracks the reduction in emotional distress as traumatic material is processed and integrated. The scale provides measurable feedback on the effectiveness of EMDR interventions, supporting both the therapist and client in gauging progress.

Takeaway

Scaling, particularly through the use of the Subjective Units of Disturbance (SUD) scale, serves as an essential tool in EMDR therapy. It facilitates the assessment, monitoring, and guidance of the therapeutic process while enhancing client engagement and self-awareness. By offering a clear and straightforward framework for clients to express their emotional distress, the SUD scale empowers individuals in their journey to healing. It allows them to track their progress and gain meaningful insight into their reactions to trauma.

This structured approach not only supports more effective treatment outcomes but also fosters a sense of control and agency in clients as they work through their challenges. By naming and rating their internal experiences, clients gain a deeper understanding of their emotional states and become more engaged participants in their own healing.

Grounding

Grounding techniques are strategies employed in psychotherapy and counseling to help clients remain grounded in the present moment, particularly during times of distress, emotional overwhelm, or dissociation (Laganiere & Bouchard, 2019).

One of the most widely used methods is the 5-4-3-2-1 grounding technique, also known as the Five Senses method. This simple but effective mindfulness exercise is commonly integrated into therapeutic settings to help individuals manage anxiety, stress, or overwhelming emotions (Doe, 2019). As part of a broader set of grounding practices, the 5-4-3-2-1 technique brings awareness to the immediate environment through sensory engagement. Other grounding methods may include body awareness, breathing techniques, tactile grounding, or interacting with the environment to re-establish a sense of safety and presence.

Instructions for the Five Senses (5-4-3-2-1) Grounding Technique:

Find a Comfortable Space

Take a Few Deep Breaths

Engage Your Senses:

Sight: Look around and identify five things you can see.

"What colors, shapes, or objects do you see?"

Touch: Focus on four things you can feel.

"Notice the texture of your clothing, the feeling of the chair beneath you, or the temperature of the air on your skin."

Hearing: Listen for three sounds in your environment.

"What sounds can you hear right now? It might be the rustling of leaves, distant traffic, or even your own breathing."

Smell: Identify two things you can smell.

"If there are smells around you, pay attention to them. If not, try smelling your sleeve or your skin."

Taste: Notice one thing you can taste.

Five Senses (5-4-3-2-1) Grounding Technique: Client Example

Counselor: You mentioned wanting to find ways to cope when feeling overwhelmed. How would you like to try a grounding exercise?

Client: (inhales deeply, exhales slowly) Yes, I'd love to try anything to help.

Counselor: Great. Keep taking a few more deep breaths. When you're ready, we'll go through the five-senses grounding strategy.

Client: Okay, I'm ready.

Counselor: First, look around and notice five things you can see. What do you notice?

Client: I see a lamp, your laptop, a green plant on the desk, a blue mug, and a picture on the wall.

Counselor: Great. Now, focus on four things you can feel.

Client: I can feel the air conditioning on my skin. I can notice my toes in my socks, my hands on my jeans, and the chair beneath me—it's pretty comfy.

Counselor: Okay. Now, listen for three sounds in the environment.

Client: I hear the hum of the air conditioner, the ticking of a clock, and my own breathing.

Counselor: Good. Next, identify two things you can smell.

Client: That's a tough one. I don't have a good sense of smell. I guess I can smell the air—it's almost like a coffee smell—and maybe vanilla hand lotion?

Counselor: Lastly, notice one thing you can taste.

Client: I can taste the coffee I had earlier.

Counselor: Great! How are you feeling now?

Client: I feel a bit more grounded, more present. It helped me focus on my senses.

Counselor: That's great to hear. Remember, you can use this technique anytime you need to reconnect with the present moment.

Takeaway

Grounding strategies, such as the Five Senses (5-4-3-2-1) method, are essential resourcing tools in therapy, particularly within the context of EMDR. These simple yet powerful techniques are designed to enhance present-moment awareness and foster a sense of safety and connection, both of which are crucial when processing traumatic memories. By intentionally engaging the senses of sight, sound, smell, taste, and touch, clients reinforce their grounding and stabilize their emotional state, thereby easing symptoms of anxiety, stress, and trauma responses.

This increased sensory awareness anchors clients more fully in their bodies, helping them avoid dissociation or states of hypoarousal. If left unaddressed, such states can significantly interfere with the therapeutic process. In essence, grounding strategies act as internal resources that empower clients to regain a sense of centeredness and presence during overwhelming moments, making the overall therapeutic experience more effective and supportive.

Window of Tolerance

The Polyvagal Theory, introduced by Steven Porges in 1994, provides a deeper understanding of the intricate relationship between the nervous system, emotional regulation, and behavior (Porges, 2001). At the core of this theory is the concept that the autonomic nervous system plays a pivotal role in how we manage stress, connect socially, and respond to perceived threats.

The theory offers valuable insights into how both the sympathetic and parasympathetic branches of the nervous system influence our emotional and physical responses to stress and trauma. Through this lens, we begin to recognize how the nervous system governs whether we feel safe, mobilized, or shut down.

Daniel Siegel (1999) expanded on this understanding by exploring the relationship between the brain, body, and mind and introduced the concept of the "Window of Tolerance." This refers to the optimal zone of arousal within which an individual can function effectively—emotionally, cognitively, and socially—without becoming overwhelmed or shutting down. When a person's emotional arousal exceeds this window, they may experience anxiety, panic, dissociation, or numbness, making self-regulation and engagement challenging.

The Window of Tolerance highlights that each person has a threshold of emotional intensity they can manage before their nervous system becomes dysregulated, triggering a fight, flight, freeze, fawn, or collapse response. Recognizing and working within this window enables clients to regulate their emotions more effectively, stay connected during therapy, and develop resilience over time.

Siegel (1999) emphasized the importance of developing positive body awareness as a foundation for emotional and psychological well-being. Techniques such as breathing exercises and grounding practices can help widen the window of tolerance, enabling individuals to handle a greater range of emotions and stress without becoming dysregulated.

Takeaway

Expanding one's window of tolerance is a crucial aspect of developing emotional stability and resilience. This involves learning to process emotions within a manageable range, without becoming overwhelmed or disconnected. By broadening the window of tolerance, individuals can improve their emotional regulation, coping skills, and relationships while also reducing symptoms of anxiety and depression.

Safe Place

Creating a safe place is a guided mental imagery exercise designed to evoke feelings of calm, security, and peace. In therapy, clients are asked to focus their attention on a mental space where they feel emotionally and physically secure. While the word "safe" is commonly used, some individuals, especially those with histories of abuse or disempowerment, may find it problematic to connect with the term. In such cases, the words "calm" or "secure" can be used instead.

Once a client is able to visualize a place that evokes positive feelings of safety or calm, they are encouraged to embody the experience, focusing on how it feels in their body and mind. If the client is unable to visualize, they might want to draw a calm place on a piece of paper or even bring in a photograph of a quiet place to refer to. With attunement, it is essential to meet the client where they are. The exercise may involve engaging all five senses to describe the space in detail: what they see, hear, feel, smell, and taste. This sensory engagement strengthens the emotional connection to the imagined place.

The concept of dual awareness is also central to this resourcing strategy. It refers to the understanding that a person can be in two places at once—mentally anchored in their safe place while also remaining physically present in the therapy room. This dual awareness creates a bridge between the inner and outer world, fostering both emotional regulation and grounded presence.

This activity demonstrates the power of the mind to visualize, sense, and internalize a secure space, reinforcing the client's awareness that they have control over their mind and body. It also helps the individual recognize that the current environment is secure enough to begin therapeutic work on sensitive issues.

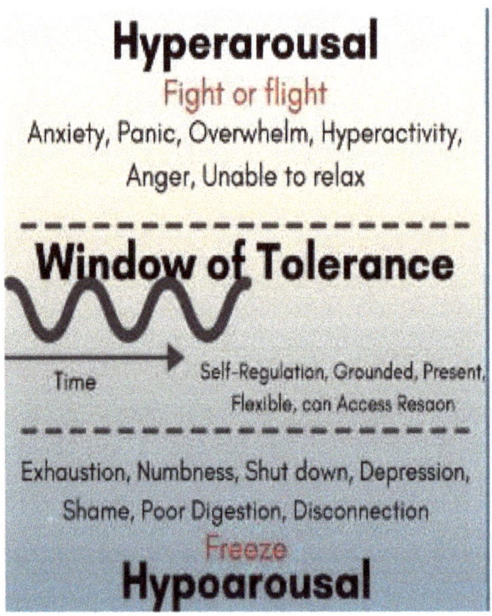

To create a calm and secure place for emotional stability and comfort, clients are guided through a visualization exercise. They are encouraged to explore the sensations and emotions they experience in this imagined space, allowing them to immerse themselves in and fully embrace the feeling of safety. Eventually, the client is asked to mentally "anchor" the safe place, holding onto its details and associated positive emotions. By naming this place, the client creates a personal and meaningful reference point that can be returned to throughout therapy for grounding and emotional stability.

Instructions to Create a Safe Place

Instruct the client to sit comfortably in a quiet and safe environment.

Ask them to close their eyes and take a few deep, calming breaths to center themselves.

Begin guiding the visualization by asking questions such as:

"Imagine a place where you feel completely safe and at ease. What does this place look like?"

"What colors, shapes, or objects do you see?"

"What sounds are present in this space?"

"Are there any smells or sensations you can notice?"

Encourage the client to engage all five senses and to describe what they feel in their body while in this space. For example:

"What feelings do you experience here?"

"What do those feelings feel like in your body?"

"Where do you feel them? How big are they?"

"Allow yourself to embrace those feelings ."

Takeaway

Imagining a calm, safe, or secure place to retreat during times of stress is a powerful relaxation and resourcing technique. By fully engaging both hemispheres of the brain—through vivid visualization, sounds, scents, sensations, and even taste—clients can calm their nervous systems, reduce anxiety, and foster a deep sense of peace and well-being. This becomes a reliable internal resource that can be accessed at any point during therapy or daily life. It is important to understand that not all clients can visualize. In that case, it is fine to have them draw a picture of a space or not to do this exercise at all. In addition, it is not wise, as we attune to our clients, to expect a client who has vast amounts of trauma to have a concept of safe. 'Safe' can be a word that triggers a fear response in them.

Securing the Space

There are times when, with attunement, we notice that a client struggles to engage with the concept of a safe place. For some, especially those with histories of trauma, imagining a "safe" place may evoke discomfort or even overwhelm. The part of the self that holds trauma may interpret safety as dangerous. This felt sense is somatic in nature. Even though the client is physically safe in the present—in your office or online session—the protective mind may still issue an automatic, maladaptive response to a perceived threat rooted in past experiences.

In these cases, the therapist—through careful observation and attunement—can choose not to introduce a traditional safe place but instead focus on securing the present space. This technique, developed by Jim Knipe, helps clients increase their sense of current safety without requiring them to visualize an external or imagined location.

Securing Your Space (Adapted from Jim Knipe)

Goal

To assist clients who struggle to access a calm or peaceful place or who are unable to let their guard down. This exercise helps clients develop the ability to secure the space they are currently in, regardless of the setting. It can be used at the beginning of any session—particularly in virtual therapy—to ensure that the client's immediate environment feels safe enough for therapeutic work.

Steps

1: Explain the Concept:

"Even though the environment may not always be completely safe, today we'll explore ways to help you increase your sense of safety, as much as possible, right where you are."

Measure Security: Ask: "How secure do you feel right now on a scale from 0 to 10, where 0 means not secure at all, and 10 means as secure as you can imagine being?"

Show the scale: 0 1 2 3 4 5 6 7 8 9 10

2. Identify Security Elements or Strategies:

Ask: "What makes this space feel secure right now?"

As the client lists each element (e.g., locked door, dim lighting, favorite blanket, presence of the therapist), use 6 to 8 slow bilateral taps to reinforce it.

3. Gauge Security with the Therapist:

Ask: "How secure do you feel with me, as your therapist, right now?"

Tap in this connection slowly and supportively, reinforcing the bond.

4. Remeasure the Security Level:

Ask: "Now, how secure do you feel for us to go forward? Is there anything else you need to feel even more secure in this space?"

Throughout the process, the therapist can attune to behavioral cues that may indicate internal discomfort, such as shifts in posture, tone, or eye contact. These subtle signs provide insight into the client's felt sense of safety.

Importantly, this exercise also supports the repair of attachment. When a person holds trauma, the experience is often one of isolation: the prefrontal cortex goes offline, and the autonomic nervous system takes over. By staying present and engaged with the client while co-creating safety, the therapist provides the client with a new experience: they are not alone, and someone is actively working with them through whatever emerges in therapy.

The Container

At the beginning of therapeutic work, it is helpful for the therapist to introduce the concept of a "container"—an imaginative or practical tool that allows clients to create a personal space for storing emotions, memories, or issues they are not yet ready to face. This internal resource provides a method for safely setting aside intrusive thoughts or overwhelming feelings during sessions, promoting a sense of control and emotional stability.

The therapist encourages the client to imagine what their container might look like. It could be a box, a vault, a sea can, a treasure chest—whatever design resonates with the client and conveys safety and strength. An essential part of the exercise is imagining that the container has a secure mechanism for opening and closing it. This feature empowers the client to control what they choose to store and when they choose to access it.

As the client visualizes this container, the counselor may ask reflective questions:

"Is the container sturdy enough to hold what you need it to hold?"

"What size does it need to be?"

"What color or texture does it have?"

"Where do you feel safest keeping it—in a room, underground, or somewhere else?"

This creative visualization supports the client's ability to compartmentalize experiences, set boundaries around their emotional space, and regain control when feeling overwhelmed.

For clients who struggle with visualization, the container can be created in a tangible form. For example, a decorated box, envelope, or jar can be used to physically hold notes, symbols, or representations of distressing thoughts or emotions. The act of writing down or drawing a worry and placing it in the container externalizes the emotion, reducing its psychological hold.

Younger clients might benefit from using tools like a worry doll, which offers a tactile and imaginative way to express and store concerns. These physical representations facilitate emotional exploration in a way that feels manageable and age-appropriate.

Instructions to Create a Container

This practice can be done either through visualization or by using physical materials.

Visualization Option:

Guide the client to sit quietly, close their eyes, and take a few deep breaths. Ask them to picture a secure container that can hold any thoughts or emotions they're not yet ready to deal with. Encourage them to notice its size, shape, color, and security features (such as locks, lids, or doors). Invite them to place unwanted thoughts or feelings into this container and mentally "lock" it.

Physical Option:

Invite the client to use a box, envelope, or bag to represent the container. They can write intrusive or distressing thoughts on slips of paper, draw images that represent emotional discomfort, or find physical items to symbolize their experiences. Once placed in the container, these items are "put away," giving the client a sense of emotional relief and containment.

The process reminds the client that they can return to the container and open it when they are ready to address its contents, on their own terms and in a therapeutic space.

Takeaway

Introducing the concept of a container at the start of therapy provides clients with a grounding tool for managing emotions and intrusive thoughts they are not yet prepared to confront. Whether visualized or physically constructed, the container becomes a symbolic and functional space for setting emotional boundaries. By reflecting on its characteristics and using it intentionally, clients reinforce their capacity for self-regulation, emotional organization, and mental clarity. For clients who find visualization challenging, the use of tangible objects, such as decorated boxes or worry dolls, offers accessible alternatives, empowering them to navigate therapy with a greater sense of control and safety.

Breathing, Diaphragmatic Breathing

Research has shown that slow, intentional breathing can have a profound effect on both physical and mental health. Studies have found that this practice can increase gray matter in the brain, strengthen the immune system, and promote a lasting sense of calm and relaxation (Kox et al., 2014; Mackay et al., 2012). Breathing slowly and steadily through the nose and out through the mouth offers numerous mental health benefits, including reduced stress and anxiety, improved mood, enhanced focus and concentration, and increased self-awareness. It can also aid in emotional regulation, help manage symptoms related to PTSD and ADHD, lower blood pressure, and improve sleep quality (Brown et al., 2013; Nascimento et al., 2019).

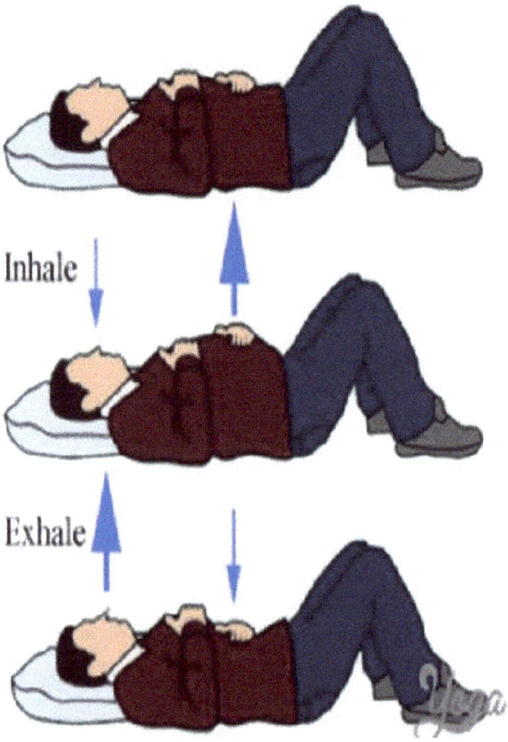

Mindful breathing allows clients to ground themselves in the present moment. Bringing awareness to the breath and practicing deep, steady breathing encourages relaxation and can reduce anxious thoughts. It activates the parasympathetic nervous system, which is crucial in calming the body's stress response and promoting internal balance. In therapy, breathing techniques can also help clients develop greater body awareness and improve emotional regulation.

There are several forms of deep breathing techniques used in therapy, including diaphragmatic breathing, box breathing, and the 4-7-8 breathing technique—all of these support controlled, elongated breathing, which helps to restore balance to the nervous system. Also known as diaphragmatic breathing, this technique is vital for activating the parasympathetic nervous system. By slowing the breath and deepening the inhalation into the belly rather than the chest, individuals can calm their central nervous system and enhance both brain and body awareness.

How to Teach Diaphragmatic Breathing

Sit/Lie Comfortably: Have the client sit or lie in a comfortable position.

Place Your Hands: Ask the client to place one hand on their belly and the other on their chest.

Inhale Deeply: Instruct them to breathe in slowly through the nose, allowing the belly (not the chest) to rise and move the hand on the belly upward.

Exhale Fully: Guide them to exhale slowly through the nose or mouth.

Some research suggests that mouth exhalation may help release tension.

Other studies recommend nasal breathing for both inhaling and exhaling to calm the nervous system and reduce anxiety (Nester, 2020).

Repeat and Demonstrate: It can be helpful for the therapist to model the breathing alongside the client for at least one minute, reinforcing the pace and rhythm.

Takeaway

Incorporating slow, controlled breathing into daily life can lead to greater mental clarity, improved decision-making, and a deeper sense of emotional and physical well-being. Regular practice cultivates a mindset of gratitude, peace, and presence. By connecting to their breath, individuals gain a reliable and accessible tool for managing stress and enhancing self-awareness.

Eye Rolls

The Eye Rolls technique blends the soothing effects of belly breathing with the stabilizing benefits of eye movement, offering a powerful tool for grounding and emotional regulation (Kabat-Zinn, 2003; Foa et al., 2010). This two-pronged approach helps individuals manage stress and anxiety more effectively without becoming overwhelmed. The synchronized pattern of deep breathing with slow eye movements supports a return to calm and enhances present-moment awareness.

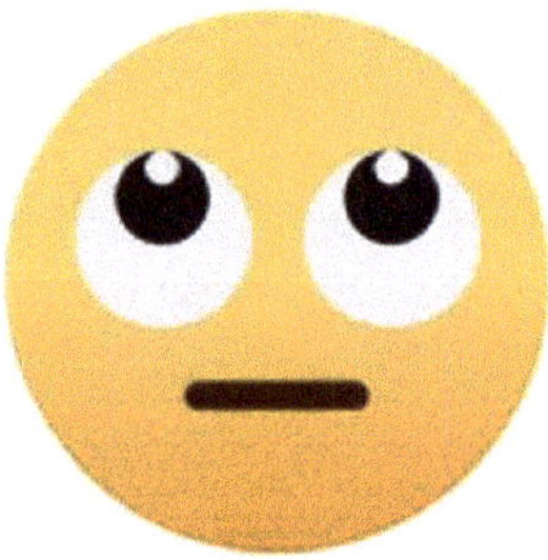

As a resourcing technique, the Eye Roll can redirect attention away from distressing thoughts and guide the mind toward balance. The rhythm of movement and breath creates a calming effect that grounds individuals in their bodies and in the present moment.

Instructions to Prompt Eye Rolls

Establish a Connection: Begin by asking the client to place a hand on their heart, maintaining a neutral gaze.

Guide Vertical Eye Movements: Instruct the client to move their eyes slowly upward as they inhale and downward as they exhale.

Coordinate with Hand Movement

Inhale: Raise your hand slowly while guiding the client's eyes upward.

Exhale: Lower your hand as the client follows with their eyes downward.

Continue Rhythmically: Repeat this pattern several times, maintaining a steady, calming pace until the client begins to feel more grounded and focused.

Takeaway

The Eye Rolls technique, used in EMDR resourcing, effectively merges breath regulation with eye movement to reduce anxiety and support emotional stability. This accessible and integrative strategy enhances emotional resilience, offering individuals a practical tool to regain composure and center themselves when overwhelmed.

Pressure Points

Pressure points on the hand, also known as acupressure points, can be utilized as a simple yet effective relaxation technique in therapeutic settings. Commonly applied in trauma work, anxiety reduction, and stress relief, this method uses light pressure on specific areas of the hand to engage the body's natural calming response (Benson & Proctor, 2010).

Tapping or gently pressing these points helps shift attention from distress to the present moment, allowing individuals to ground themselves physically and emotionally. The combination of tactile sensation and mindful breathing promotes calmness and emotional containment.

Instructions to Use Pressure Points

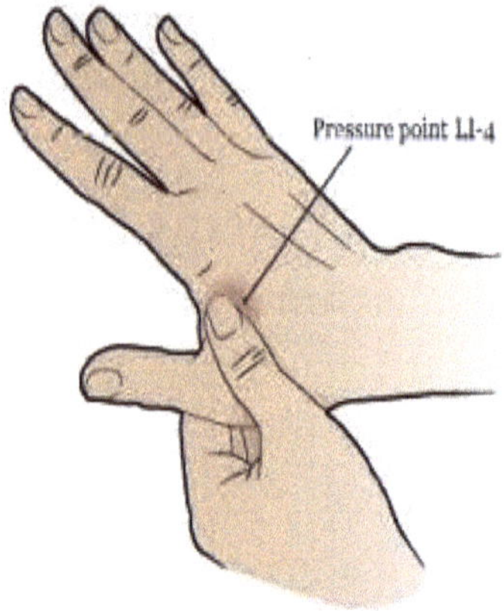

Locate the Pressure Points: Identify the space between the thumb and index finger or the center of the palm.

Apply Gentle Pressure: Using your thumb or finger, apply steady pressure to the chosen point.

Breathe Deeply: Encourage the client to take slow, deep breaths while focusing on the sensation of pressure.

Maintain the Pressure: Hold for 2–3 minutes while continuing to breathe deeply and slowly.

Release Gently: After holding, slowly release the pressure and allow a few moments to notice the shift in a physical or emotional state.

Takeaway

Stimulating pressure points can be a powerful way to support emotional regulation. This technique activates the body's innate response to stress, promoting relaxation, reducing anxiety, and helping clients ground themselves in the present moment (Benson & Proctor, 2010). It is an accessible and adaptable strategy that can be used independently or in conjunction with other resource allocation tools.

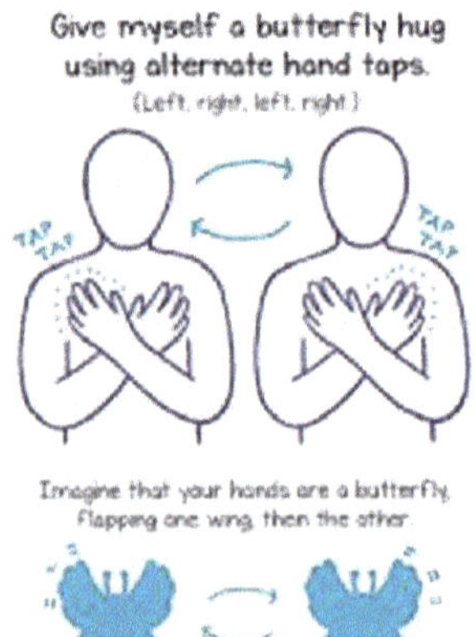
Give myself a butterfly hug
using alternate hand taps.
(Left, right, left, right)
TAP TAP
TAP TAP
Imagine that your hands are a butterfly,
flapping one wing, then the other.

The Butterfly Hug

The Butterfly Hug is a self-soothing technique used in EMDR therapy that promotes emotional regulation through gentle, bilateral stimulation of the body (Jarero & Artigas, 2024). Designed as a grounding tool, this method can be used independently or during sessions to reduce anxiety, calm the nervous system, and soften the emotional impact of distressing memories.

This technique engages both hemispheres of the brain by using rhythmic, alternating hand movements. It helps interrupt the brain's ability to maintain intense emotional responses to difficult memories, reducing their vividness and emotional weight. The bilateral stimulation also activates calming responses in the body, increasing the production of feel-good hormones like serotonin and endorphins, which support relaxation and a sense of safety.

Instructions for the Butterfly Hug

Cross Your Arms: Place your arms across your chest so that each hand rests on the opposite shoulder or closer to the collarbone—whatever feels natural and comfortable.

Position Your Hands: Your fingers and thumbs should point upward, mimicking the wings of a butterfly.

Close or Soften Your Eyes: You can close your eyes or keep them gently open while focusing on a neutral spot in front of you.

Begin the Movement: Start gently alternating taps between your hands, simulating the fluttering wings of a butterfly. Keep the rhythm slow and steady.

Breathe Deeply: Practice abdominal breathing by inhaling slowly through your nose and exhaling either through your nose or mouth.

Observe Without Judgment: While tapping, notice what comes up—thoughts, sensations, images, sounds, or feelings. Simply observe without trying to change, judge, or push anything away. Imagine these experiences drifting by like clouds.

Takeaway

The Butterfly Hug is a powerful and accessible technique that combines physical movement with mindful awareness. It empowers individuals to manage overwhelming emotions, calm their bodies, and reduce the emotional intensity of troubling memories. Whether used as part of EMDR therapy or as a standalone resourcing strategy, the Butterfly Hug supports emotional safety and grounding by engaging both the mind and body (Jarero & Artigas, 2024).

Walking

Walking is a natural, repetitive motion that helps engage both the body and brain. As each foot alternates from side to side, the movement creates bilateral stimulation, activating both hemispheres of the brain in a rhythmic pattern (Lutz, 2015). This pattern stabilizes the central nervous system and supports emotional regulation, making walking an accessible and effective resourcing strategy (Hassett & Tully, 2021).

Our bodies are designed for movement, and walking serves as a built-in mechanism for self-soothing and mental clarity. This movement facilitates the release of endorphins, which naturally improve mood and reduce feelings of anxiety or distress. Additionally, walking supports cognitive and emotional balance by promoting coordination between the left and right sides of the brain.

In this way, walking is more than just physical activity—it becomes a form of moving meditation, encouraging individuals to focus on the present moment, regulate their breathing, and calm their minds. This mindful movement supports the integration of physical and emotional awareness, fostering a sense of groundedness and mental clarity.

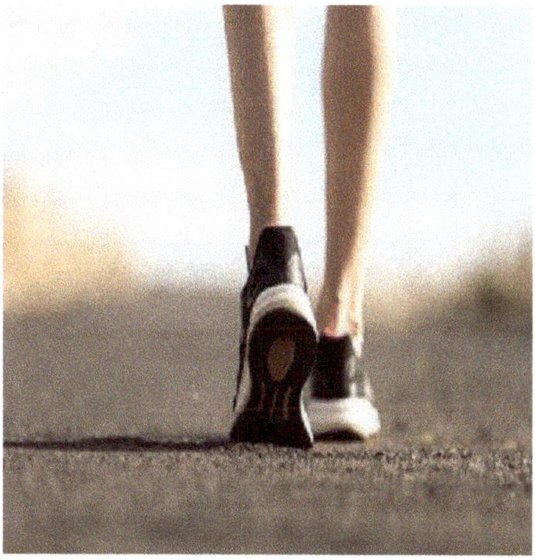

Instructions to Walk as Resourcing

Find a Comfortable and Safe Space: Choose a quiet, open area where you can walk without distractions or obstacles.

Set a Gentle Pace: Walk slowly and steadily, maintaining a pace that feels relaxed and comfortable.

Breathe and Relax: Before walking, take a few deep breaths—inhaling through your nose and exhaling through your mouth—to ease tension in your body. It is also acceptable to incorporate counting into this exercise. Counting in breath for seven and out for eleven.

Be Aware of Your Surroundings: Pay attention to what you see, hear, and feel as you walk. Use your senses to stay connected to the present moment.

Observe Your Thoughts: As thoughts enter your mind, allow them to pass without judgment. Gently return your focus to the sensation of walking.

Maintain a Consistent Rhythm: Walk for about 10–15 minutes, keeping your breathing calm and your heart rate steady.

Takeaway

Walking is a simple yet powerful way to promote emotional regulation and mental well-being. Through bilateral stimulation and rhythmic movement, it helps restore balance to the nervous system, reduces stress, and supports mindfulness. As a grounding resource, walking serves as a natural and effective way to navigate emotional challenges and enhance resilience.

Movement

The body holds on to emotions—especially those tied to sadness, fear, or trauma—within the nervous system (Scaer, 2005). This stored emotional energy can lead to physical manifestations such as tension, anxiety, or chronic stress. When these emotions are not processed, they may result in emotional numbing or disconnection (Hart, 1993), making it more difficult for individuals to recognize, experience, and regulate their emotions.

Releasing this stored energy is essential for healing and restoring the body's natural rhythm. Movement-based practices help unlock the nervous system's capacity to reset and return to a state of balance.

According to Van der Kolk (2014), engaging the body through movement is a vital step in trauma recovery, as the body often retains memories that the mind may not be able to articulate.

Somatic Experiencing (SE), developed by Peter Levine (2017), emphasizes gentle movement, awareness, and breathing as methods for helping the nervous system discharge pent-up energy. These movements need not be complex—they may involve stretching, swaying, or slow, mindful gestures—anything that fosters awareness of the body and encourages the release of tension.

Takeaway

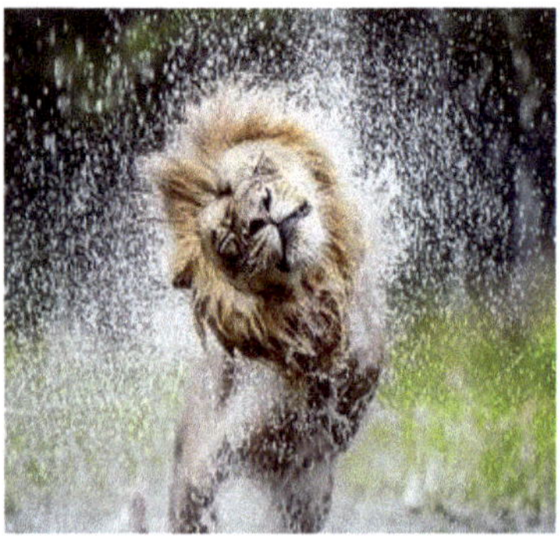

Movement is a core element in processing stored emotional energy. By gently activating the body through breathing and somatic techniques, individuals can begin to release trauma, reduce emotional distress, and restore a sense of safety and control. Integrating movement into therapy supports the reconnection of body and mind, enabling deeper emotional healing and long-term resilience.

A technique employed in Somatic Experiencing (SE) and other trauma-informed approaches is known as Movement by Shaking. This method aims to release stored emotional energy and tension by encouraging gentle, rhythmic body tremors (Levine, 2017). Shaking engages the nervous system's natural ability to discharge stress, restoring a state of balance and calm. It is beneficial for clients dealing with unresolved trauma, anxiety, or chronic stress, as it offers a physical pathway for emotional release.

By fostering a sense of safety and enhancing bodily awareness, this technique allows individuals to reconnect with their physical selves and reduce emotional numbing, a standard protective response to trauma. Clients often report feeling lighter, more grounded, and more connected to their emotions after engaging in this practice.

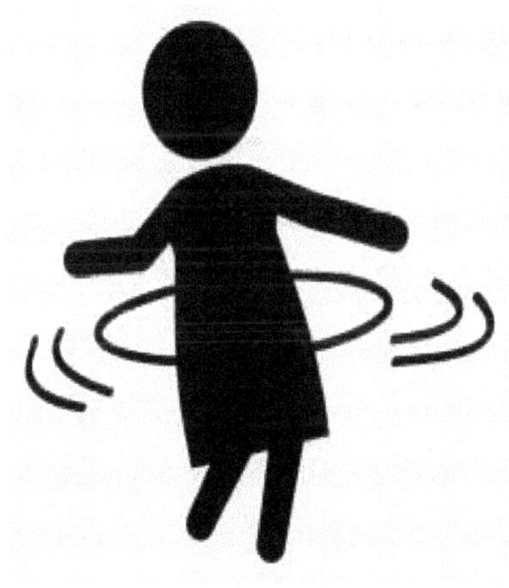

Example of Movement by Shaking

Find a Comfortable Space: Stand with your feet shoulder-width apart to ensure balance.

Begin with Breath: Take a few deep breaths, inhaling through your nose and exhaling through your mouth, allowing your muscles to relax.

Start Small: Begin by gently shaking your hands.

Expand Gradually: Slowly incorporate movement into your arms, shoulders, and then gradually into your torso and legs. Let the motion be free and natural.

Optional Intensity: You may gently increase the intensity if it feels right, staying mindful of your limits.

Set a Time: Continue the shaking for about 5 minutes or until you feel ready to stop.

Cool Down: Gradually slow the movement. Return to stillness and take a few calming breaths.

Observe: Notice any changes in how your body feels. Allow your system to settle before moving on.

Takeaway

Emotions that have been suppressed or unresolved may appear as physical symptoms such as tension, anxiety, or emotional shutdown (Draijer & Langeland, 2010). These symptoms can interfere with the ability to remain grounded, which is necessary for effective EMDR therapy (Shapiro, 2018). Movement, such as shaking, supports the body's innate ability to release this energy, helping clients regain emotional presence and readiness for deeper therapeutic work. It is a simple yet transformative technique that fosters emotional clarity and resilience.

IDEA Framework

The IDEA framework, developed by Saj and Mete (2025), offers a structured and flexible model for integrating multiple therapeutic approaches. The acronym stands for:

- **I** – Identify the issue
- **D** – Determine the initial approach
- **E** – Engage in integration
- **A** – Assess and evaluate progress

This framework is advantageous when working with clients in EMDR therapy who may benefit from additional resourcing strategies or when a single approach proves insufficient.

The IDEA framework supports a client-centered, collaborative process, allowing therapists to adapt techniques in real-time and tailor interventions to individual needs. This flexibility is especially valuable in the context of attunement and resourcing, where different clients may respond to different strategies based on their emotional readiness, regulation, and history.

Saj and Mete (2025) emphasize the integration of bilateral stimulation, movement, breathing techniques, emotional regulation, and neural connectivity to support whole-person healing. Their research suggests that layering modalities—such as combining physical movement with emotional processing—can deepen therapeutic outcomes and help clients develop lasting tools for regulation and self-care.

The IDEA Framework in EMDR Therapy

The IDEA framework is a systematic approach that helps prepare clients for their treatment and encourages collaboration between clients and clinicians to find effective healing methods. It is instrumental in counseling and EMDR discussions, providing alternatives when traditional resourcing techniques fall short.

Saj and Mete's (2025) research emphasizes the importance of resourcing techniques, including bilateral stimulation and movement, in helping clients establish a sense of safety. As previously noted, clients must feel secure and capable of engaging in EMDR therapy for it to be effective. There are numerous avenues for future research in this area, and clinicians must invest time in the preparation phase to attune to their clients. Having a diverse set of resourcing strategies and the awareness of the IDEA framework readily available is vital for effectively supporting clients.

Conclusion

This chapter outlined various resourcing techniques crucial for preparing clients for the eight stages of EMDR therapy. These strategies aim to enhance emotional and physical regulation, fostering the client's ability to engage effectively in the therapeutic process. Key topics included the importance of regular check-ins to assess emotional states and the development of emotional awareness. We discussed the use of scaling to communicate emotional readiness and the practice of grounding techniques to promote present-moment awareness.

Furthermore, the chapter explored the concepts of the window of tolerance and polyvagal theory, providing a framework for understanding optimal arousal levels.

Specific resourcing techniques covered included:

- Visualization of safe and secure places
- Diaphragmatic breathing for relaxation
- Physical strategies such as eye rolls, pressure points, and butterfly hugs to manage emotional intensity
- Movement-based approaches, such as walking, are used before and during EMDR sessions.

Integrating the IDEA framework into these discussions underscores the systematic approach it represents in preparing clients for their treatment. It encourages collaborative exploration between clients and clinicians to discover effective healing strategies. This framework is particularly beneficial in EMDR and counseling contexts, offering structured alternatives when traditional resourcing techniques may prove insufficient.

Research by Saj and Mete (2025) reinforces the significance of bilateral stimulation and movement in fostering a sense of safety in clients. As emphasized, clients must feel secure and supported to benefit from EMDR therapy.

With an array of resourcing strategies and a clear understanding of the IDEA framework readily accessible, clinicians can effectively support clients during the preparation phase. The incorporation of these insights strengthens the foundation of stability and self-regulation necessary for clients to navigate the therapeutic process with greater ease and resilience.

Moreover, a wealth of opportunities for future research in this area remains, highlighting the ongoing evolution of best practices in EMDR therapy.

Section 3
Integrating Attunement into the Eight Phases of EMDR

Attunement Across Phases 1–2: History Taking and Preparation

In this section, we transition from foundational knowledge to a more in-depth exploration of how *attunement* can be refined and applied within each of the eight phases of EMDR therapy. This is not simply about following protocol—it is about learning to sense, feel, and respond with precision to the unique psychological and physiological needs of the client. We begin with the History and Treatment Planning phase, which is not just about gathering facts but about establishing a relationship grounded in trust, curiosity, and care.

Attunement in the History and Treatment Phase of EMDR Therapy

When a client first walks into the room, their healing does not begin with the protocol—it starts with a feeling. And that feeling is safety. Emotional safety. Relational safety. Neurobiological safety. The first doorway into that safety is the question:

"What is your goal in therapy? What matters to you most?"

This isn't just an intake checklist—this is an invitation. It's the beginning of attunement. The answer they give may be spoken in words, or it may be whispered through posture, breath, silence, or eye movement. Our role is not to rush past it but to *witness* it.

Beyond Words: Tracking the Client's Nervous System

Attunement in this stage means listening with all our senses. It means being present enough to notice:

- How the client's breathing shifts when a particular topic comes up
- The subtle tension in their jaw or the fidgeting in their hands when they recall a memory

- Whether their eye contact holds or drifts away when talking about a parent or a partner
- If their body stiffens when asked about goals or expectations

Each of these is data, but more importantly, each is a signal that tells us where to tread gently and where to offer space. These cues are invitations to slow down, check in, and ask:

"How is it for you to share this with me right now?"

The Myth of Neutrality

There is a misconception—especially among new therapists—that neutrality means being still or detached. But for many clients, especially those with complex trauma, this clinical stillness can echo abandonment, disinterest, or even threat. The absence of warmth is not neutral; it's *noticeable*. And it can replicate early attachment ruptures that brought them to therapy in the first place.

The client is not just hearing our words—they are *feeling* our nervous system.

- If we are calm, they feel safe.
- If we are anxious, we brace ourselves.
- If we are flat, they may retreat.

Trauma survivors are often exquisitely sensitive to micro-signals. A tightening in the therapist's jaw, a shift in posture, a delay in response—all these may be read, rightly or wrongly, as messages. Therefore, part of attunement here is self-awareness. Before we can attune to our client, we must attune to ourselves.

Mirror of the Past: The Therapist as Attachment Figure

When we ask a client to recall past trauma, we are often asking them to return to memories of feeling unseen, misunderstood, or alone. If we enter this space with a distant, overly professional demeanor, we unintentionally reinforce the very wounds they came to heal.

Attunement means being a *regulated*, *present*, and *responsive* human being. It means making micro-adjustments:

- Slowing our voice when they speed up
- Leaning in when they pull away
- Naming the tension when the room goes quiet

It also means knowing when to step back and let silence do its work, or when to validate with warmth:

"That sounds incredibly heavy. And you've carried it for so long."

Attunement Is the First Intervention

Before any tapping or eye movement, before targets or timelines, attunement *is* the first therapeutic tool. When done well, it tells the client:

"I see you. I'm with you. And you don't have to go through this alone."

This sense of being seen—fully, nonjudgmentally, and with compassion—is what begins the work of repair.

In the following chapters, we will explore how this same depth of attunement continues through each subsequent phase of EMDR: Preparation, Assessment, Desensitization, Installation, Body Scan, Closure, and Re-evaluation. We will offer clinical examples, somatic cues, and relational markers that help therapists stay aligned, responsive, and effective in every step of the journey. Because EMDR is not just about *what* we do—but *how* we do it—with attunement as our guide.

Overt and Covert Manifestations of Symptoms

To fully understand the client's needs, we must conduct a biopsychosocial interview. This approach emphasizes the importance of actively listening to clients as they recount their life experiences and share their perspectives. Through this process, we identify "targets"—specific events or circumstances that significantly impact their daily lives.

It is good to consider that there are basically two types of trauma: trauma of commission and trauma of omission. Commission is just that... something happened that has a noted meaning, usually negative. We understand what it is; however, we may not understand why it happened. The trauma of omission is just that – traumas that occurred because something didn't happen. It may be that a parent is unable to care for a child. It may be that a sibling is very ill and the parents need to tend to the sick child, leaving the client to their own devices, whether perceptively or actually. It may be that the parent or caregiver does the best they can with the circumstances that surround the client. And with omission, things that needed to happen did not happen.

Sometimes a client will appear with overt behavioral displays that "just won't quit." Everything is safety sensitive (some people call these folks borderline personality disordered, which, for sure, has a bad connotation). The clients who come to us with this presentation are likely to have attachment wounds and are actually doing the very best they can with a maladaptive adaptive pattern. It is imperative to "dig deep" and look for the cause, not the symptoms.

It's vital to note that most individuals do not seek therapy due to a single distressing event. Instead, they often arrive at our doors after a multitude of issues, events, or challenges have compounded, leading them to realize that assistance is necessary, typically triggered by a single acute incident.

While some may equate the biopsychosocial approach with merely gathering historical data, it includes a richer, more nuanced understanding of the client's emotional landscape. Attunement plays a crucial role as we observe both overt and covert behavioral cues that reflect their emotional state. Clients may exhibit a range of manifestations, from overt expressions, such as tears or laughter, to more subtle indicators, including fidgeting or changes in posture.

Many clients might not fully understand their emotional responses. They may display "innie" behavior, withdrawing inwardly, which can be perceived as shyness, or "outie" behavior, acting out or defensively vocalizing their distress. Regardless of the outward expression, these behaviors often serve as protective responses to perceived or real threats.

As we delve deeper into history-taking, we look for age-appropriate reactions that reveal the timeline of disturbances in the client's life. A client who demonstrates childlike behaviors or struggles to articulate feelings may indicate that their distress originates from experiences before they had the cognitive tools to process or express them, often dating back to formative years, sometimes even prenatal experiences.

Exploring Early Influences

It's essential to recognize that some experiences may even stem from events that occur during gestation. For instance, a child born to a mother who suffered multiple miscarriages may be predisposed to anxiety or other emotional disturbances due to the maternal environment during pregnancy. While the child may not consciously comprehend this pain, they could internalize a felt sense of fear simply from existing in that context.

When clients first arrive for therapy, they are often in the process of determining whether they can trust us with their most vulnerable aspects. Our attunement to their needs is vital in this early stage. In EMDR therapy, while we adhere to a structured protocol, therapists can recognize the importance of flexibly responding to the unique needs of each client within that framework.

Individualized Approach to Therapy

Every client presents a distinct narrative. Our approach must reflect this individuality rather than fitting them into a pre-existing mold. Attunement becomes particularly critical when encountering neurological diversity among clients, where cognitive processes may vary significantly. This variation underscores the necessity of calibrating our understanding of each client's mental processes during the history-taking phase.

During this process, we actively encourage clients to articulate their feelings, identifying where those sensations manifest within their bodies or minds. By acknowledging their "system," we foster a more holistic understanding of their experiences, both physical and psychological.

Recognizing the role of attunement during the biopsychosocial phase also plays a part in attachment repair. Trauma often leaves individuals feeling isolated and vulnerable, leading to physiological responses such as shallow breathing or activation of the fight, flight, freeze, or fawn response. In these moments, specific brain structures become less active, and emotional responses arise from deeper neurological pathways that are triggered by perceived (or real) threats.

Our role as therapists during this initial phase is to create a safe and supportive environment where clients can narrate their experiences without fear of judgment or reactivation. Many may struggle to voice traumatic events aloud, akin to trying to hide spoiled food in a refrigerator. The subject is frightening and often repulsive, making it difficult to confront, and, therefore, the maladaptive adaptive skill of avoidance comes into play.

Sensitivity and Listening Skills

As clients begin to open up, it's essential to approach sensitive topics with care, encouraging them to share just enough of their experiences to feel validated without overwhelming them. Clients might want to divulge every detail of their trauma, but our focus should remain on their emotional state and physical responses as they recount their narratives.

During the biopsychosocial interview, we gather foundational historical information while avoiding delving too deeply into trauma processing. Our goal is to understand what has transpired, when it occurred, and how it affected them. Before venturing further into therapy, we must ensure that clients feel safe and equipped to manage their emotions.

As our initial meetings conclude and we have gathered preliminary information, we will develop resourcing strategies—tools and techniques that prepare clients for more in-depth discussions. The goal is to establish a therapeutic environment that reiterates our role as allies in their journey. Clients should understand that we walk alongside them, rather than being immersed in their emotional turmoil.

Neurobiology of Trauma

The connection between trauma and the brain provides valuable insight into our clients' experiences. When discussing the brain's mechanisms, particularly regarding how trauma interacts with mental processes, we might explore models of the autonomic nervous system. These models typically describe two types of arousal: hyperarousal, associated with fear and anger, and hypoarousal, linked to numbness and dissociation.

Traumatic responses primarily stem from complex interactions within specific brain structures. The brainstem plays an essential role in how we respond to trauma, and understanding this can enhance our therapeutic strategies. For instance, the superior colliculi, locus coeruleus, and periaqueductal gray are key players in our emotional and defense mechanisms during trauma responses.

Upon encountering unexpected stimuli—such as a sudden noise or an alarming situation—the superior colliculi initiate orienting movements in response to the novelty. This reflex is not only limited to threats; it also encompasses a broad range of stimuli.

The relationship between these neurological responses and body awareness can guide body-based trauma therapies. Recognizing how the brainstem structures react during trauma can help both therapists and clients understand the physiological components of their experiences.

In conclusion, this highlights the importance of attunement, a biopsychosocial approach, and an understanding of the neurobiological processes underlying EMDR therapy. Engaging clients sensitively, encouraging them to explore their feelings, and recognizing their unique narratives are vital steps in facilitating healing and growth within the therapeutic landscape.

Attunement and Preparation in EMDR Therapy

In the second phase of EMDR therapy, the focus is on preparation. At this stage, we assist the client in preparing for therapy. We assess where they are in terms of understanding their feelings, possessing self-knowledge, and recognizing their strengths as they prepare to process the traumatic events that led them to therapy.

There are several key considerations that we must remain mindful of to effectively prepare the client for EMDR processing. These include:

- Addressing issues of competency and responsibility
- Exploring the origin of negative cognitions
- Preparing within the context of dissociation

Consideration in the Preparation Stage of EMDR

Preparation is the stage of "getting the client ready". Ultimately, the goal of preparation is to foster a sense of safety, control, and emotional resilience, enabling the client to embark on the trauma processing phase with confidence. In EMDR therapy, the preparation stage is crucial for establishing a solid therapeutic foundation, particularly when addressing themes of existence, competence, and responsibility.

When a client expresses feelings of inadequacy, such as saying, "I'm not good at doing my job," this sentiment often reveals deeper fears and survival instincts that could be traced back to formative life experiences (also known as attachment wounds).

During this preparation phase, clinicians focus on helping clients unpack the implications of their fears and examine the roots of their negative beliefs. When a client articulates concerns about job competency, it is crucial to explore the emotional weight behind their statement. Questions like "What does it mean for you if you're not good at doing your job?" and "What's your biggest fear about it?" serve to illuminate the survival mechanisms at play, such as the anxiety surrounding financial stability and family support.

This reflective process encourages clients to confront and articulate their feelings about competency, thereby fostering self-awareness and emotional resilience, key goals of the preparation stage of EMDR. Furthermore, understanding the origins of these beliefs can help clients recognize how past experiences, including those related to upbringing, culture, or neurological diversity, contribute to their current self-assessments.

For instance, a client who has faced the challenges of feeling out of place in conventional settings may have internalized a belief of incompetence. As the clinician probes these beliefs, it may lead to insights about how experiences from childhood continue to influence the client's self-perception and performance in their current job.

By addressing these layers during the preparation stage, clinicians create a safe space for clients to explore their feelings and discover their strengths. This process not only prepares clients to deal with traumatic memories but also fosters a sense of empowerment and capability, effectively bridging the gap between their past experiences of incompetence and their present potential for growth.

By integrating the exploration of competency and responsibility into the preparation stage of EMDR therapy, clinicians can help clients establish a solid foundation of self-awareness and resilience that will support them as they navigate the trauma processing phases of their treatment.

The Dual Aspects of EMDR

EMDR has two dimensions: the cognitive "head" aspect, which encompasses the techniques we learn, and the emotional and felt sense "heart" aspect, which guides our attunement to the client. The heart aspect fosters curiosity, allowing us to connect with the client. In contrast, the head aspect organizes thoughts to create a structured treatment plan. We need both the EMDR head and heart to make sense of what the client is bringing to therapy.

Float Back Technique

The "float back" technique involves asking clients to hold an image in their mind alongside a negative cognition (belief), like *"I'm not good enough."* The clinician encourages them to allow their mind to drift back to an earlier time when they felt similarly and to describe the first scene that comes to mind.

This process works through the unconscious mind, encouraging clients to recall feelings that might not be at the forefront of their consciousness. The clinician might ask, "What do you say to yourself when you feel this way? What does it mean for you to feel that you aren't good enough?"

Shapiro urged clients to "float back" and find the very first representation of events that are encoded as trauma. It is wise to note that many of the events that happen to our clients are non-verbal. This may mean that the event(s) took place before the mind could make cognitive sense of them. Therefore, it is possible that the client may not be able to come up with a thought or an image of the earliest event. It could be that the event (target) may be a somatic feeling, a felt sense. Know that we can process the somatic feeling event with just as much efficacy as an event that has concrete information.

In floating back, it is also wise to consider that some trauma happens in the womb. For example, a fetus can experience the angst and anxiety of the mother while gestating. In that case, we can still process those memories using an EMDR protocol, *When There Are No Words* (Sandra Paulson). There is always a way, an adaptation to the basic protocol that will enhance processing if we are attuned to the client's needs.

Focusing on Self-Referencing

The negative cognitions we explore are always self-referential. For example, rather than stating *"Life has no worth,"* a client might say, *"I am worthless,"* indicating a personal belief rather than commenting on life itself.

How we get to having the client realize the negative belief(s) may be just as simple as saying, after we do a biopsychosocial review, "Because all of those things happened to you, what did it make you believe or think about yourself?"

Adaptive cognitions (beliefs), which counter negative beliefs, need to be grounded in reality. For example, if a client feels *"totally helpless,"* we might frame the positive cognition as *"I'm empowered to cope."* Or it could be *"I do the best I can, regardless."* This reframing helps the client resonate with something more realistic and achievable.

Importance of Realistic Positive Cognitions

Positive cognitions should always be adaptive and realistic. For example, while *"I'm always okay"* might not resonate with situations that need resolving, *"I'm empowered to cope"* does. This distinction is crucial in effectively processing negative beliefs. The positive cognition must realistically resolve all trauma-based events, including the thoughts, feelings, and somatic underpinnings that exist stored in the neurological network of the client, regardless of the age at which the client experienced a traumatic event.

Addressing Competency Concerns

If a client expresses feelings of incompetence, they may worry about hurting others in their life. They often assume undue responsibility for outcomes that are not solely within their control. This self-imposed pressure can hinder therapeutic progress. For example, it is unrealistic for a child to maintain order in a chaotic setting. A child can only do the best they can given the circumstances.

This competency concern can hinder the processing of traumatic memories. Think of it like this: if a client feels—or has been led to believe for all the right reasons—that they have no competency because they have not been able to process a traumatic event, then the neurological network picks up that feeling and can slow down or stop processing. The small brain then resorts to maladaptive adaptive ways of dealing with matters. This can result in a system stall or shutdown.

Resilience Amidst Traumas

In dealing with historical trauma or systemic oppression, it's crucial to validate clients' experiences while highlighting their resiliency. For instance, ask them if they did their best in a challenging environment. The goal is to help them recognize their inner strength, despite the challenges of external circumstances.

Throughout this process, the focus should always be on personal strength and resilience. By exploring positive cognitions and beliefs and acknowledging the challenges they faced, we can guide clients toward a deeper understanding of their worth and capabilities.

Preparation in the Context of Dissociation

When preparing clients for therapy, particularly those experiencing dissociation, several crucial factors must be taken into consideration. Most importantly, clinicians must hold faith in their clients' capacity to heal.

Important mental content is either available to awareness or is not. However, in reality, there is often a degree—a spectrum—of mutual awareness between different ego states, also known as parts or aspects of self. In another point in our manuscript, we will explore psychological defenses such as avoidance, idealization, shame, or addiction. These are all mental activities (perhaps partially conscious or potentially unconscious) that prevent complete trauma processing but exist to reduce the impact of distressing memories or disturbing awareness of parts of the self.

Defenses are often maintained by positive affect, for example, the relief that comes with successfully avoiding an unpleasant memory or the satisfying feeling of believing oneself to be superior to others. The effectiveness of these defenses is diminished by focused sets of bilateral stimulation (BLS). The internal healing dialogue becomes especially useful in integrating mental states that are initially dissociated.

Establishing Trust

The first step involves fostering trust—not only in the clients' potential for healing but also in the clinicians' own abilities. Trauma therapists should rely on their instincts while utilizing evidence-based modalities such as EMDR, Internal Family Systems (IFS), ego state interventions, and somatic therapies to address complex trauma. Attuning to the client is essential; clinicians must cultivate a sense of calm within themselves before they can effectively support clients who may be dysregulated, agitated, or emotional.

Understanding Internal Systems

To assist clients, it is vital to understand their internal systems and how they experience dissociation. It's essential to acknowledge that dissociation is not a conscious choice; rather, it serves as a protective mechanism that helps individuals remain safe during overwhelming situations, whether real or perceived. Our role is to observe how clients manage their safety and when they (their system) feel the need to dissociate.

Welcoming Resistance

Resistance to treatment is a natural response, especially for clients with protective parts or aspects of self—whether identified through IFS or ego states—that fear losing their ability to shield themselves. It is essential to reassure clients that none of their behaviors is inherently "bad." These behaviors have often been vital for their survival over the years.

Many clients with complex trauma struggle to remain present, often feeling disconnected from their experiences. As therapists, it is our responsibility to help them recognize their current reality while acknowledging that trauma is part of their past. We should consistently seek permission and feedback from clients, being attentive to any shifts in their emotional state, and allowing them to participate in the conversation actively.

The Importance of Patience and Celebration

Patience is essential. Clients with extensive trauma histories may be hesitant to revisit painful memories until they feel safe and assured in our ability to navigate this journey with them. We should celebrate even the smallest achievements during sessions, such as moments of increased awareness, a sense of grounding, or the ability to remain present while discussing complex topics.

Whether clients exhibit "innie" behaviors (dissociating) or "outie" behaviors (acting out), it's essential to recognize that both represent protective states of consciousness.

Addressing Pre-Verbal Trauma

When working with trauma—particularly early attachment trauma—many experiences are often pre-verbal. Expecting clients to articulate their experiences may not be realistic, especially if their frontal cortex was not fully developed to process these memories. Clients may respond with uncertainty or say, "I don't know," when asked about their past. This response can indicate a somatic sensation that lacks a straightforward narrative.

Pre-verbal trauma is often not remembered, but it is frequently expressed in the person's most comfortable—or most uncomfortable—mode of interacting with others, and perhaps in their general attitude (positive or negative) about life. Early experiences sometimes determine the feeling tone of specific, important questions:

- *What kind of world am I living in?* (safe or unsafe, interesting or boring, friendly or unfriendly)
- *What kind of people are in my world?*
- *What kind of person am I?* (Am I mainly aware of myself and my needs, with the needs of others less important? Or am I highly tuned in to what others are thinking and feeling because that awareness expands my world?)

A very young child automatically and non-consciously makes assumptions that begin to answer these questions, and then those assumptions are carried into later ages, which are better remembered in therapy. Early preconscious learning may be a key element in why a client struggles today to feel happy, prosperous, or secure.

In other words, comprehensive therapy sometimes involves helping a client become aware of their own object relations patterns, the origins of those patterns, and alternative object relations patterns that could be more satisfying to them.

In these situations, we should avoid pressuring clients for answers that don't resonate with them. Instead, we can invite them to describe their bodily experiences. If these sensations feel overwhelming, we must approach the topic with care and gentleness.

One effective strategy is to use third-party observational techniques, encouraging clients to observe their experiences from a distance rather than being immersed in them. This technique—often referred to as *distancing*—may involve asking clients to visualize their experiences as if they were watching a movie or witnessing a child who resembles them or their situation from their childhood.

Preparation in the context of dissociation requires a multifaceted approach: fostering trust, understanding clients' internal systems, welcoming resistance, and recognizing the complexities of trauma. By celebrating small wins and being patient, therapists can provide essential support while guiding clients through their healing journey.

This understanding details the preparation phase of EMDR therapy, focusing on attunement and readiness. The core objective is to establish a safe and resilient foundation for trauma processing by helping clients understand their feelings, recognize strengths, and explore the origins of negative beliefs, particularly those related to competency and responsibility. Clinicians employ techniques such as the float-back method to access early traumatic memories and facilitate self-referencing, thereby emphasizing the development of realistic, adaptive, and positive cognitions.

We stress the two dimensions of EMDR—cognitive and emotional, which are crucial for understanding client needs. Addressing dissociation requires building trust, understanding internal systems, accepting resistance, and practicing patience while celebrating progress. Adaptations for pre-verbal trauma involve focusing on somatic sensations and using distancing techniques to explore memories gently. Ultimately, the preparation stage aims to empower clients, enabling them to confront trauma with confidence.

Phases 3-6: Assessment, Desensitization, Installation, and Body Scan

Attunement and Assessment in EMDR Therapy

This chapter will examine additional considerations in the assessment phase of EMDR, highlighting the significance of attunement during this stage.

The assessment phase in EMDR is crucial for establishing a successful therapeutic process. During this phase, the therapist and client collaborate to pinpoint the specific memory or issue the client wishes to address. A detailed assessment that employs a target sequence plan is imperative for effectively organizing the therapeutic work.

The target sequence plan is simply a map—a map that the therapist and client use to understand the inner world of the client and work with to process events (past, present, and future) to a place of balance in the neurological system. This process involves identifying the emotional, cognitive, and sensory aspects associated with the client's experiences. Such a structured approach is essential in EMDR, as it creates a solid foundation for the effective processing of traumatic memories, ensuring that therapeutic interventions directly address the most significant effects of those memories.

The client is encouraged to detail the distressing memory as thoroughly as possible, sharing any associated emotions, thoughts, and physical sensations. The therapist assists the client in identifying the *negative cognition* (NC), which represents the negative belief or thought pattern linked to the memory, and the *positive cognition* (PC), which is the more constructive belief or thought pattern the client wishes to adopt.

Additionally, the client rates their level of distress on a scale from 0 to 10 (SUD: Subjective Unit of Disturbance) both before and after the session to monitor changes in their emotional state. This information enables the therapist to assess the suitability and timing of proceeding with EMDR processing and to tailor the treatment plan to meet the client's specific needs.

Developing a Target Sequence Plan

A key concept in understanding the neural underpinnings of EMDR therapy is the concept of *synaptic plasticity*, which refers to the brain's ability to reorganize and adapt its neural connections throughout life. Research has shown that every time two neurons fire together, a new synaptic connection is formed, and when they fire together repeatedly, that connection becomes stronger. This concept is often described as *"neurons that fire together, wire together."*

This idea is closely related to another concept known as *Hebbian learning*, which states that *"neurons that fire together, wire together."* This phrase, coined by Canadian psychologist Donald Hebb in 1949, essentially means that the more neurons communicate with each other and fire together, the stronger the connection between them becomes. Over time, this repeated communication can lead to the formation of neural pathways that are more efficient and automatic, allowing the brain to process information more quickly and easily.

This process can be both beneficial and detrimental. On the one hand, synaptic plasticity allows the brain to learn new information and adapt to changing circumstances. On the other hand, when maladaptive or traumatic memories are stored in the brain, they can become deeply ingrained in the neural network and can be difficult to change.

EMDR therapy aims to tap into this process of synaptic plasticity to help individuals reprocess and integrate traumatic memories. By activating the neural pathways associated with a traumatic memory, EMDR helps to weaken the connection between the neurons and rewire the brain with new, more adaptive information. Over time, this can lead to a reduction in symptoms and an improvement in overall mental health.

Target Sequence Planning

The objective of target sequencing is to gather information in an attuned manner that will facilitate the processing aspects of EMDR therapy. The goal of the target planning process is to create a roadmap for the reprocessing phases of EMDR. A roadmap is essential because, if we are working with a client in a manner that responds to their needs, then we must create a map in order to know where we're going.

We begin by identifying significant emotions, cognitions, and sensations, as well as their origins. It's important to note that emotions, sensations, and cognitions are merely representations of underlying information, issues, or targets that have been predominantly affecting the client's life.

Regardless of the case formulation process, the goal is to develop the target sequence plan and identify the corresponding negative and adaptive positive neural networks. This outline provides the foundation for treatment—and not only for EMDR but for most other psychotherapy models as well.

It's also important to understand that, although we are discussing EMDR therapy, creating a target sequence plan is highly beneficial in other types of therapy as well.

Sometimes a client will come in with what we call a *single presenting complaint*, and we want to identify that concern while also exploring its associated symptoms, dominant emotions, sensations, and cognitions. We can ask the client to *float back* to earlier times when this issue was experienced and even look ahead to future events where it may resurface.

The key to attunement is understanding that the presenting issue is not isolated—it's a doorway into the client's larger history and the neurological network that has accumulated meaning over time.

As clinicians, we must remain attuned to the full spectrum of what has transpired, not just the surface-level complaint.

We notice that there is a chronological timeline to the client's pieces of information, and what we want to do is create a timeline of the disturbing experiences. When the client discusses these experiences and shares information, it's best not to ask for too much detail, as that can trigger them in a potentially dysregulated way.

Again, we'll be clustering the information by emotion, sensations, and beliefs. We will then prioritize the clusters and develop a written target sequence plan that guides us through past, present, and future information.

Oftentimes, people will organize this on a timeline or use a *genogram*. When we use a genogram, we are developing a historical program—a biopsychosocial map—and using it to find potential targets from the past (epigenetic) that may be influencing the present.

A genogram is especially useful for what we call *epigenetic targeting*. Epigenetic targeting refers to identifying how certain emotional or behavioral patterns may have been passed down through generations. This often includes emotions, sensations, and beliefs related to events that never actually happened to the client directly but occurred in the lives of caregivers or other family members.

A key aspect of a genogram is to identify the historical information, allowing the client to trace their responses to life elements that can be dysregulating.

Sometimes, a client presents with multiple symptoms, and we need to prioritize them accordingly. If those symptoms are distinct, we can create separate target sequence plans for each. Interestingly, we may find that the beliefs are similar or even identical across different events. Activities that cause dysregulation can produce similar symptoms, even when the events themselves differ in nature.

When a recurring trigger occurs, a client may report several incidents that appear to be related to one another. These might include physical or verbal attacks, car accidents, or repeated losses. In such cases, the client's response to each of those events may follow a similar emotional and sensory pattern.

You can ask the client, "When you think of these incidents, do they bring up the same emotions, sensations, and beliefs?" Based on that, you can create a target sequence plan that focuses on the negative cognitions and themes. List each experience that resonates with those core beliefs, sensations, and emotions. It is also important to note that it is not essential to list every single event that one has experienced during a lifetime. We may seek out the highlights of their experience, and when we process, since we are examining synaptic plasticity, these events listed will link with others and be processed, regardless of whether they are known and listed.

If the sensations, emotions, and beliefs are different, it's also possible to create a map that incorporates these various elements. The mapping of targets can be a creative and unstructured process that grows from deep attunement to the client. The way a client expresses what has happened to them is unique and should not be met with any preconceived expectations from the clinician.

Some clients are visual. Others are auditory, somatic, or even olfactory in how they report experiences. If the targets are from early in life, there may be no words for how the client feels or thinks.

In fact, when you engage in this mapping process, the client retains control in drawing out what is on their mind while you assist in making the connections. These connections are vital—they reveal the ongoing ways a client adapts to situations that have long been problematic.

Considerations: Attunement and Assessment

For the sake of understanding the client's whole experience, we build what is known as a *target sequence plan* based on the presenting issue. This plan helps us examine the neural network and identify the connections between what is happening in the present, what has happened in the past, and what may happen in the future. We begin by identifying the issue, symptoms, triggers, behaviors, and somatic experiences the client wishes to work on. These targets can be rooted in the past, present, or even anticipated future. Targets can be real or perceived, or metaphorical.

As we explore these areas, we are mindful not to overwhelm the client. Instead, we attune carefully, asking about emotions and sensations they are feeling or expecting to feel, without pressuring them or pushing too deep before they are ready for processing.

We then ask the client to discuss what these emotions and sensations mean to them. What we're truly looking for is the client's verbalization of the emotions as a *negative cognition or belief*. According to Francine Shapiro, *a belief is the verbalization of a cognition.* In practice, we often find that these negative beliefs are familiar to the client and function as a kind of keystone belief that has shaped their self-perception over time.

At this stage, we may use direct questioning or *float back* and *float forward* interventions to identify the three prongs of the target sequence plan:

- Past memories
- Present triggers
- Future anticipated events or situations

We do this while following the client's lead.

Through direct questioning or by reflecting on past experiences, we can identify earlier memories that connect to the present cognitive themes and emotional patterns. When possible, we work to identify the *touchstone memory*—the earliest remembered experience or feeling state that embodies the negative belief. However, it's essential to stay attuned: clients may not always recall their earliest memory. If they say, *"I don't know,"* we can gently explore *how they are aware of the negative belief, even if it is not accompanied by a clear memory,* and make a note of that. Not all memories present themselves in words.

When traumatic experiences occur before the frontal cortex is fully developed, the memories may be stored somatically rather than as coherent, named cognitive memories. In these cases, clients are more likely to describe feelings or body sensations than full narrative memories.

Clients may also come in with present triggers—events or stressors currently happening in their lives that they want to address. We know from neurobiology that the brain stores similar events over time, building patterns of emotional and physical responses. The presenting issue may simply be the latest iteration of a long-standing neural pattern.

Similarly, future triggers can be identified through forward-looking techniques or direct questions. We ask clients to imagine a future situation where the same feelings or sensations might arise, then observe what they believe about themselves in that context.

Once we have gathered all of this information, we transfer it onto a piece of paper—our *target sequence plan.* The format of the plan is flexible, as long as it clearly outlines the past, present, and future targets and triggers that contribute to the client's distress. The goal is to make the internal landscape visible and structured, both for the clinician and for the client.

Finally, it is helpful to ask: *"What do you believe about yourself because all of these things happened to you?"* The answer often reveals a core negative cognition that may span multiple events. Then follow up with: *"Given everything that's happened, what would you rather believe about yourself?"* This helps the client identify a *positive cognition*—one that is adaptive, grounded in reality, and emotionally resonant. This contrast between the negative and positive beliefs forms a critical foundation for EMDR processing.

Farming for Positive Belief and Building Resilience

The question *"What would you rather believe?"* opens the door to identifying a positive belief or internal strength the client may hold without even realizing it. In our work, it is very wise to intentionally *"farm"* for that belief. When we farm for it and engage in *personal resourcing* (which we will cover in more detail later), we activate a positive belief system that has always been present, though often buried beneath maladaptive patterns.

Clients develop *maladaptive-adaptive* coping mechanisms—responses that once served a protective purpose but may have now become ineffective. These patterns take over, and the mind, in its effort to stay safe, continues to recycle those responses. However, as time goes on, these strategies no longer serve the client well. Life becomes increasingly unmanageable, and they seek therapy as a result.

By introducing personal resourcing that draws from a positive belief, we help the client recognize that they do, in fact, possess adaptive strategies for coping—ones that are healthier and more sustainable than their maladaptive defaults. Developing and accessing these adaptive ways of responding to life's challenges can shift the client's entire trajectory toward long-term resilience and emotional regulation.

Defining Internally Located Positive Beliefs

It's essential that the positive belief is *internally referenced*—that is, the belief must reflect the client's own self-referenced sense of identity and capability, not dependence on others. For example:

- *"I'm good in the world regardless"* points to an internal truth that holds even when external circumstances change.
- In contrast, *"I'm good because my mother treats me well"* is externally referenced. It relies on another person's behavior to validate self-worth and would not be suitable for EMDR processing simply because it depends on another person for wellness.

Confirming Resonance Across the Network

Once we have outlined the negative neural network, we must confirm that the *positive cognition* resonates across all the incidents identified. This step ensures that the belief is stable and robust enough to serve as a foundation for the client throughout the process.

We then identify recent times when the client successfully accessed or embodied that positive belief. This becomes the foundation of personal resourcing. It opens the corridor for the client to process from within an *adaptive network*, rather than continuing from the same maladaptive framework that has previously failed them.

Adaptive Information Processing (AIP) Framework

The AIP model rests on the idea that the amygdala encodes the past as if it were the present. People respond today based on how they were treated, what they internalized, and how their past experiences shaped their nervous systems. Human beings are hardwired to seek safety and connection. Any threat—real or perceived—activates emotional encoding, and the stronger the perceived threat, the stronger the emotional and neurological imprint.

Therefore, when a client arrives in your office and expresses overwhelming distress about current events, it is wise not to allow emotional flooding to take over the session. When a client exhibits excessive emotion, they may be outside their *window of tolerance*, which puts them at risk for dysregulation.

Instead, attune to the underlying reality: the more expressive and intense the current emotion, the more likely there's a *stacked accumulation* of past unprocessed experiences that are surfacing now through the current trigger.

Implicit vs. Explicit Memory

From the AIP perspective, we recognize that *presenting issues* activates implicit memory networks. The distinction between implicit and explicit memory is critical here:

- **Implicit memory** is not conscious. It may manifest as a feeling, a bodily sensation, or a somatic experience with no clear cognitive origin.
- **Explicit memory** is conscious. It's a piece of information, an image, or a narrative that the client can recall and describe.

Both implicit and explicit memories carry equal weight in shaping behavior and emotional responses. Cognitions are often the *verbal expression of implicit emotions and sensations*.

So, when we ask, *"What meaning have you drawn about yourself because of what happened?"* we are trying to access that core negative cognition—the belief that has shaped the client's internal world. It is also helpful to listen to the client's concern *from the perspective of the child within them*, because many of these beliefs originate in early developmental stages when the frontal cortex was not yet equipped to make sense of the world rationally.

By acknowledging this childlike lens, we deepen our attunement and lay a foundation for more compassionate, effective processing in therapy.

Children internalize. For example, they may feel or say, *"I'm unlovable because my parent don't hug me."* Cognitions and beliefs are self-evaluations. And what that means to the client—when we attune to them—is that the client is telling you what they believe about themselves based on experiences or information or behaviors that other people have actually indicated to them. And often, those indications are not about the client themselves, but about the situation the client is in.

Cognitions and beliefs can be very dramatic at times, and the more dramatic they are, the earlier the encoding occurs. We aim to investigate the nature of a client's negative cognition and its underlying origins. You might say stuff like, "*What does it mean if you're not good enough? What does it say about you? What's your greatest fear if you're not good enough?*" Now, the origins of negative cognition or belief could be rooted in survival, responsibility, or competency.

Survival could mean *that if I'm not good enough, I'll be abandoned and die.*

Responsibility, *if I'm not good enough, others will be hurt.*

Competency: *If I'm not good enough, I am a failure.*

So, when a child, a teenager, or an adult is told over and over again that they are in a deficit situation, their system will take that on as truth and begin to use a compensatory strategy.

Now, there is something we want to look at, and that is normalizing the adaptations the client has made to survive. Individuals from a variety of cultural backgrounds, or those with attachment or developmental trauma, are forced to be externally focused in order to survive and excel in adverse environments. If we are attuning to the client, we also want to examine their adaptive mechanisms and what they have done to survive or thrive (including both maladaptive and adaptive behaviors).

It can be challenging to help them maintain an internal perspective when they frequently encounter external threats. Oftentimes, we will have a client come into our office who, at the time of their meeting with us, is still in a situation that is adversarial to some degree for them.

Now, those threats or adversarial situations can be encoded as part of a target or something that's happening in the present, which will exacerbate the effects of past experiences.

When examining culture, we must also consider—and this is part of the attunement process—why this is happening to this particular client. *What does it mean to this client?* And to be very honest with oneself as a clinician, that maybe my culture—the clinician's culture—is very different than the client's culture. And it is so that we can ask questions to clarify.

For example, If a person comes from an Asian culture, there may be a cultural belief that children must take care of their parents and grandparents when they need help.

Well, that can sometimes work for our client, and sometimes it doesn't. However, when we examine our client, who comes to us and discusses the demands of their parent, it becomes clear that the parent's cultural persuasion may differ from that of the client. Now, if the client has moved here from another country, another part of the world, we want to ask those questions. Not that we're going to lay blame or wag a finger at a parent or a grandparent who needs help, but we have to understand what the distress level is by attuning to the client rather than attuning to a situation where we, clinically, might feel it's unreasonable. Now, chances are it may be irrational, but the cultural aspect comes into play and must be regarded and held in high esteem.

Cultural and generational considerations might include, again, that *my family expects me to provide financially for my siblings and parents.* The negative cognition or belief could be that *I'm responsible for everything,* and this may be the cultural norm in the family. However, it may be unrealistic in the context in which the client is.

Now, a positive belief could be that *"I can take responsibility and still have my needs met,"* or *"I can take responsibility and still learn how to meet my own needs."* The client might state, *"The world's not safe for me."* The negative belief might be that *I'm not safe.* Ongoing discrimination may be in play due to race, gender identity, sexual orientation, religion, or other such matters.

And basically, that could be very true. The client may still be embroiled in situations because of their race or their gender, their sexual orientation, or their religion, which brings a lot of angst into their life just because.

Now, the positive aspect of this is that *I can learn ways to keep myself as secure as possible and do the best I can under the circumstances, even if I'm in a dangerous place.*

Well, you could also simplify it by saying *I do the best I can, regardless,* and carry on with the work of processing.

Attunement During Sessions

When clients express doubts about their capabilities, it's crucial to effectively attune to their emotions. Encourage self-reflection by asking questions such as, *"What advice would you give someone else in your situation?"* This external perspective can help clients recognize their strengths and resilience.

Understanding Presenting Issues and Symptoms

Our focus should be on the presenting issues or symptoms from a neurological standpoint, particularly by utilizing the Adaptive Information Processing (AIP) model, rather than solely adopting a psychological perspective.

Present Triggers

Present triggers can activate both past explicit and implicit memory networks. The cognitions or beliefs that emerge from these triggers often serve as verbalizations of the implicit emotions and sensations being experienced.

Attunement and Emotional Responses

Attunement involves actively listening to clients as they verbally articulate their triggered emotions and sensations, rather than concentrating exclusively on the sensations themselves in that moment. These cognitions often reveal how individuals assess themselves, typically shaped by childhood experiences.

For instance, if a client states, *"My dad always called me stupid,"* you might respond with, *"I want you to recognize that those words do not define you. If your dad called you stupid, what do you believe about yourself?"*

The client may respond in a manner that resonates—or doesn't. If they reply, *"Well, I'm a frog,"* you might find that confusing. However, if they say, *"I guess It just means I'm stupid,"* you can probe further: *"What does that imply about you? Is it possible you feel inadequate? But is that really the truth?"*

Sometimes, underlying beliefs may be rooted in deeper fears, such as the fear of being so inadequate that it threatens their sense of survival. Here, we engage in a questioning process driven by curiosity rather than confrontation.

In therapy sessions, attuning to clients' emotions is essential, especially when they express doubts about their capabilities. Encouraging self-reflection through questions like, *"What advice would you give someone else in your situation?"* can help clients recognize their strengths and resilience, simply because if they can imagine that there is something in their strengths-based beliefs that they know and maybe have not considered. It's essential to examine presenting issues and symptoms from a neurological perspective, utilizing the Adaptive Information Processing (AIP) model to understand how present triggers activate past memory networks, thereby eliciting cognitions that reflect underlying emotions.

Active listening is key during this process, allowing clients to articulate their feelings and self-assessments shaped by past experiences. For instance, if a client mentions an experience of being called "stupid" by a parent, prompting them to explore their beliefs about themselves can lead to insights into their self-worth and deeper fears of inadequacy. This questioning process should be rooted in curiosity rather than confrontation, fostering a supportive therapeutic environment. It is worth noting that curiosity is a keystone of attunement and attachment repair.

Identifying Negative Beliefs

When clients come to us, they often discuss current events and seek solutions for how these events impact their emotions. However, we know that these present triggers often activate past implicit memory networks. As we begin to connect with the client, we need to look beyond their surface narratives to uncover the origins of these triggers.

These triggers lead to cognitions or beliefs that verbalize both implicit and explicit memories. The client's presentation is intertwined with various memories, sensations, and emotions. These cognitions or beliefs typically represent self-evaluations that were formed during childhood or within significant relationships.

It's essential to note that the more dramatic the symptoms, the earlier the underlying beliefs may have been encoded, regardless of whether these memories are explicit to the client. As we explore the deeper meanings behind the client's beliefs and their origins, we start to develop a target sequence plan.

When we investigate the origins of a client's beliefs, we aim to uncover underlying causes rather than merely addressing symptoms. Often, a client's behavior reflects the symptoms of those underlying causes. For instance, if a client expresses a belief of *"not being good enough,"* it may sound like a negative belief, but it is not entirely so.

To understand this better, we might ask, *"What does it mean to you if you're not good enough?"* or *"What is your greatest fear related to that belief?"* If the roots are tied to survival, responsibility, or competence, their responses may vary. For example, a client might say, *"If I'm not good enough, people will leave me."* This can lead us to investigate further what they felt they needed to prove to their caregivers to prevent abandonment.

Regarding responsibility, a client could express that if they aren't good enough, someone might get hurt. Often, clients believe that failing to act responsibly can lead to harm for others, even though they might not have had control over the events themselves. Generally, people do the best they can with the tools at their disposal.

When clients express feelings of inadequacy tied to competence or responsibility, it suggests they hold misplaced beliefs about their abilities. Questions such as *"When you feel that way, what do you say to yourself?"* or *"Who taught you to see yourself this way?"* can help unravel these thoughts.

These negative cognitions need to focus on the *self* rather than external situations. For example, a harmful belief like *"I'm worthless"* describes a global view of the self, while *"I'm worthless to my father"* is more situational. Emotionally charged beliefs often evoke strong feelings when recalled.

We will create a target sequence plan that incorporates both negative and positive beliefs. Writing this plan down will help the client recognize cognitive matches and mismatches. The client will be able to reflect on their past experiences in conjunction with their current self-perceptions. This process aims to establish a goal: to link and integrate past negative experiences into the present neural network.

Typically, we compile a chronological list of significant events in our clients' lives, from early childhood to the present. We also include their concerns about the future, as these anxieties often serve as valid beliefs or events that shape their behaviors. Anxiety, for example, frequently stems from past experiences or feelings, experienced in the present, but always directed toward future possibilities.

It's crucial for us to be attentive to our clients, looking beyond their behavioral responses to identify the origins of their concerns.

Several common themes help us better attune to the client and trace the sources of their beliefs. For instance, if a client discusses survival or existence, they are likely referencing memories from early childhood that have accumulated over time. They may express core beliefs such as *"I've made a mistake," "I'm unwanted," "I'm invisible,"* or *"My needs don't matter."* These reflections often reveal feelings of abandonment or betrayal, indicating experiences from a young age that shaped their self-perceptions.

As clients progress through life, they may also express feelings of powerlessness or helplessness, as well as a need for control. The feelings of survival and existence may even precede verbal communication; as clients begin to understand their lack of control, they may articulate these feelings more clearly.

As they develop further, they might express a sense of responsibility—that they must be responsible for everything. For example, a child in a parentified role, where the parents are unable to fulfill their responsibilities, may feel they are accountable for their own well-being, even though it is impossible for a child to meet adult expectations. This can lead to feelings of failure, incompetence, and inadequacy.

Clients may also wrestle with feelings of worthlessness, believing they are unlovable, unimportant, or that their needs do not matter. They may feel they don't fit in or belong. These negative cognitions tend to emerge later in life when the frontal and prefrontal cortices are more developed, allowing for complex thought patterns about self-image.

In their teenage years, clients might experience feelings of vulnerability, doubt their judgment, and worry that they don't fit in or feel trapped. Often, less responsible parenting can inadvertently create environments that foster a sense of vulnerability in children.

Identifying Positive Beliefs

Next, we turn our focus to identifying positive beliefs or cognitions. A positive cognition is adaptive, realistic, and capable of countering negative beliefs. It should emphasize a strong internal locus of control, meaning that a person should feel okay without relying on external validation (e.g., *"I'm fine regardless..."*). It is actually true regardless of what the client has been led to believe through experience or lack of understanding.

These positive beliefs should resonate as solutions to past disturbances in the client's experience. For instance, if a client with a history of trauma feels powerful, that belief might not be appropriate. Instead, a more fitting belief would be, *"I can control what I can,"* recognizing that a child cannot control an adult or perpetrator, but can make choices to keep themselves safe, even if that safety, over time, becomes maladaptive.

When examining positive beliefs, it is essential to consider their relationship to negative ones. As we document these beliefs, we must ask ourselves if the client can truly resolve their feelings with the proposed positive belief. If not, we might need to refine it further.

To identify a constructive or positive belief, we might ask questions like, *"How would you handle this situation differently?"* or *"What advice would you offer a friend facing the same issue?"* This encourages clients to adopt a more adaptive perspective while managing their difficulties.

For example, if a client feels *"totally helpless,"* a positive counter might initially be *"I'm powerful."* However, given their circumstances, that may feel unrealistic. Instead, a belief like *"I'm empowered to cope regardless of what's happening"* may resonate more effectively, allowing them to acknowledge their capacity to deal with their situation, regardless of what others in the periphery might do or not do.

Our goal is to develop positive beliefs that address the client's symptoms, resolve past experiences, provide support for their inner child, and prepare them for future challenges. This means considering the client's past, present, and future experiences to foster positive adaptations. Once a positive cognition is established, we can ask the client to identify three or four recent situations in which they successfully experienced their positive belief, often in their day-to-day life. Incorporating these examples into our target sequence plan reinforces their adaptive network.

Clients often overlook their positive experiences, especially during challenging times. By prompting them to recall instances where they successfully utilized their positive beliefs, we help them build a resource for better managing their thoughts and emotions across different contexts.

Personal Resourcing

Personal resourcing is just that. We have reviewed various ways of resourcing individuals, exploring numerous ideas on helping our clients self-regulate. All of these approaches are essential for the client to feel in control and foster the ability to meet their regulatory needs, both in the therapeutic context and in life in general.

Personal resourcing involves working with the client's positive neurological network to enhance the adaptive neural pathways in ways that are familiar to them. Werk and Kiessling have worked with what they call a *wheel of adaptive resources,* in which they ask the client to think of a positive belief about themselves and then recall times when this belief was experienced as true.

Now, the experiences that the client will note are usually not about the negative issues. For example, if the positive belief is *"I am good regardless,"* then we would be asking the client to think of times when they were or are good. It's the little things that count here. Meaning, maybe they are good at making macaroni and cheese, and it brings them great delight to do so. It can build feelings of competency and agency in our clients when we suggest that the same feelings and understandings that occur in the little things in their lives will create a positive neurological impact on the bigger things. Hence, asking them to notice the tiny things is more important than with slow bilateral stimulus, which involves "putting them in," meaning building an adaptive neural network that can operate within the system.

What does that feel like? How does it make you feel to know a competency? We can ask the client how they know that the state of well-being actually exists, noting that they may respond with a thought, a feeling, a somatic representation, or a mental image. Any representation is correct as long as the client can define it, and further, it is self-referential.

When this state is determined, a few slow BLS passes will "install" it in the positive adaptive network. The importance of this exercise lies in the fact that the adaptive network, as opposed to a maladaptive network, needs to be online to help process the negative issues. Again, the maladaptive/adaptive network takes over in the absence of a better, more adaptive way to do things in the client's life. While the maladaptive/adaptive network once worked for the client, it may no longer be helpful and can even hinder the client's progress toward wellness.

When using this technique, consider the small things that bring us joy and make us more aware of ourselves in a supportive and healthy light. These events are often small and seen as inconsequential, but when we add the slow BLS, we enhance their meaning and efficacy in the most positive ways, allowing for greater ease in reprocessing.

In this chapter, we have explored the critical role of attunement during the assessment phase of EMDR therapy. By collaborating with clients to identify specific memories or issues they wish to address, therapists create a structured target sequence plan that acts as a roadmap for therapeutic work. This plan not only establishes a clear pathway through the client's past, present, and future experiences but also facilitates the processing of traumatic memories in a way that reflects the client's emotional, cognitive, and sensory realities.

By actively uncovering negative cognitions and their origins, therapists can identify maladaptive patterns that may be hindering a client's well-being. This process involves a delicate balance of questioning and exploration, encouraging clients to connect with their inner narratives without becoming overwhelmed.

Moreover, as we develop positive beliefs alongside negative ones, we empower clients to acknowledge their strengths and resilience in overcoming past adversities. By fostering a strong internal locus of control and recognizing successful application of positive beliefs in recent experiences, clients are equipped with the tools to navigate their emotional landscapes more effectively.

Phase 4 – Attunement and Desensitization in EMDR Therapy

In EMDR, Phase 4—the desensitization phase—aims to help clients process distressing memories and reduce the emotional charge associated with them. This phase is where clients work to minimize the negative feelings and thoughts linked to their trauma memories. The therapist employs bilateral stimulation (BLS), such as but not limited to eye movements, tapping, hand-held tappers, or auditory tones, to facilitate this process. The goal is to enable the client to maintain dual awareness, keeping one foot in the present while accessing past traumatic memories.

In the desensitization phase of EMDR processing, it is crucial to prepare for each client's unique needs, as not all clients can engage in full EMDR processing, which activates the entire neurological network. This phase involves managing the negative neural network while ensuring that the positive neural network is developed enough to support the client without triggering maladaptive coping mechanisms. Clients must have foundational stabilization skills, such as grounding and affect management, and should not be actively suicidal or self-harming. Maintaining dual awareness of past and present without significant dysregulation is essential for effective processing. Clients must also be able to shift between negative and positive affect states, and screening tools can help assess their stability.

Additionally, the timing and setting of EMDR sessions should be tailored to each client's specific circumstances, particularly when working remotely or within time constraints imposed by insurance or other factors. The clinician's guidance in BLS is essential, and clear communication, pacing, and adaptability to individual client needs are vital for successful outcomes.

Phase Four of EMDR therapy—*desensitization*—is crucial because it allows clients to reduce the distressing feelings and thoughts associated with trauma memories. Many clients who come in familiar with EMDR typically refer to this phase. As clinicians, we provide *dual attention stimulus*, which involves engaging one foot in the present and the other in the past, through bilateral stimulation methods such as eye movements, bilateral tapping, auditory BLS, or other techniques that stimulate both the left and right sides of the brain.

If we notice that the client can work with full EMDR processing, the bilateral stimulus needs to be fast enough—approximately two laps per second—to create distraction. Each set should last at least 20 seconds and yield a possible minimum of 30 laps of stimulation. *Attunement to the client's nonverbal cues is vital during this process.* We closely observe their breathing patterns, facial expressions, and any other physical manifestations of their internal state. Clients may exhibit signs like flushed cheeks, shifting body language, or involuntary movements, indicating their emotional and physical reactions to the traumatic memories being processed.

During this phase, the language we use must be attuned to the client's understanding; phrases like *"take a breath"* or *"notice that"* help shift attention back to the present moment without requiring a detailed narrative of their trauma. Instead of asking clients what they feel, which could trigger more intense emotional responses, we encourage them to briefly describe what they notice or experience, understanding that each client may process internally in unique ways. Some might visualize images, while others may rely on auditory cues, sensations, or even somatic responses.

Questions during processing should remain general, prompting clients to consider *"What is emerging for them"* rather than focusing directly on their feelings. Clients often link related memories throughout this neurological processing; therefore, it is essential to keep our expectations reasonable and avoid directive comments that could interfere with their experience.

We continue this cycle of processing until clients report no change in their disturbance levels, as indicated by a SUD score. By gauging SUD levels, we can determine the depth of processing and decide whether to return to the original target event or continue with more rounds of bilateral stimulation.

This careful monitoring helps ensure that clients remain within their window of tolerance, as some may struggle to process all aspects of their experiences without becoming overwhelmed or dysregulated. In such cases, we can adapt the duration of bilateral stimuli or utilize *restricted processing techniques*, keeping the therapy focused and manageable while still working toward the goal of *installation* in Phase Five.

Considerations with Desensitization and EMDR

However, there are additional considerations within the desensitization process. Some of the key factors discussed below for the desensitization stage of EMDR include client readiness, the occurrence of medical conditions, and the complex nature of trauma. Most people can eventually be worked with in EMDR therapy, but it's crucial to evaluate their window of tolerance, stability, and specific needs. This includes considering how they engage with therapy, as well as their ability to stabilize before we begin processing.

When assessing a client's readiness for EMDR, several key considerations come into play. Firstly, it's essential to evaluate whether the client possesses basic stabilization skills, such as grounding techniques and affect management, which we have likely already worked on in Phase 2. To confirm retention of these skills, it's a good idea to review them and possibly conduct a "demo" of EMDR processing by asking the client to think of a mildly bothersome, everyday event (with a SUD of around 4) and utilizing a protocol like *Critical Incident Desensitization* (CID) (Kiessling) *(see last chapter for adaptations to processing)*. Additionally, a thorough risk assessment is necessary to determine if the client is actively suicidal or engaging in self-harm, such as cutting. If this is the case, it's crucial to prioritize further stabilization and developing a sense of self before proceeding with EMDR processing, as the client's immediate safety and well-being take precedence.

When considering the implementation of EMDR therapy, it is essential to evaluate various medical conditions that may impact the treatment process, including seizures, brain injuries, and vision issues. For clients with seizure disorders, either epileptic or non-epileptic, it is crucial to ensure they are stable and under medical supervision. Clinicians should inquire about the client's medication regimen, including the duration of seizure freedom, and take precautions by avoiding eye movements or light bars that could trigger seizures during therapy. It is also advisable to have safety measures in place, such as having the client set their car keys on a table to prevent driving in the event of a seizure and establishing a safety contact for transportation after the session should the need arise.

Clients with traumatic brain injuries may also benefit from shorter sets of processing to prevent headaches. Individuals with eye issues, such as migraines or those using progressive lenses, may find tapping or auditory forms of bilateral stimulation more tolerable than visual stimuli. For pregnant clients, particularly those in high-risk situations, the focus should generally be on resourcing until stability is confirmed, while the general consensus is that normal pregnancy does not contraindicate EMDR processing.

Furthermore, medication considerations are vital, as certain substances—particularly benzodiazepines—can inhibit the effectiveness of EMDR. Clinicians should address any active substance use or addiction, emphasizing the importance of the client's choice and the understanding that addiction can be a maladaptive-adaptive response to overwhelming circumstances. It is crucial to approach these situations with empathy and attunement, recognizing that removing substances too abruptly might lead to cross-addictive behaviors or exacerbate existing addictive patterns before EMDR processing is well-established. Adapting EMDR protocols for clients with addiction-related issues is critical for ensuring their safety and the therapy's efficacy.

Preparation for EMDR Processing Phase 4

Ensure informed consent about the EMDR approach as part of the treatment plan. Discuss the specifics of the target sequence plan, explain the bilateral stimulation concept, and confirm the client's comfort with proceeding.

Stop Signals

It is essential to establish a stop signal to ensure client safety during processing. This signal should be distinct from verbal expressions of distress related to the content being processed. We might encourage the client to use a clear hand signal to indicate that they want to stop processing. This gives the client agency and control in the process.

Process of Desensitization

Aspects of Targets and Target Selection

In Phase Two, we prepared for EMDR processing. Now, what we have to know about processing, in terms of attunement to the client, is that not all clients can do what Francine Shapiro called *full EMDR processing.* Full EMDR processing engages the entire neurological network, as opposed to potentially targeting a single area.

The negative neural network can be (and usually is) stacked, and there can be issues and experiences that are not immediately apparent. By doing full EMDR processing, we potentially start to stir up what we might call *the pot.*

What we need to be sure of is that the *positive neural network* is sufficiently developed to, in a certain way, compensate for what arises in the negative, without causing the client to autonomically switch into their maladaptive or adaptive ways of dealing with issues.

What we're going to be doing is processing the negative neural network with the help of the positive, and we're going to consolidate the negative issues Into the adaptive or positive neural network.

Now, there are, as you may know, a few things to remember here. The client needs to have basic stabilization skills, meaning grounding and affect management, which we've already accomplished earlier in our meetings with the client.

We want to be sure that the client is not actively suicidal or self-harming. We want to be sure that the client has the ability to maintain *dual awareness*—to have one foot in the present and one in the past—without significant dysregulation.

There is a difference between significant dysregulation and a client experiencing, feeling, and having sensations about what has happened to them. *Dysregulation,* or *significant dysregulation,* is when the client cannot contain how they're feeling and does not have the ability to have a foot in the past and a foot in the present. This might mean that the client experiences the target—which is actually an event in the past—and does not perceive that they are in the present.

The client must have the ability to shift between affective states, transitioning from negative feelings to positive feelings. If we are to use any screening devices, such as the DES, the ACEs, or potentially the MID-60, we can get an idea of whether the client is able to stay present—that is, not dissociate to a great degree—in order to process the information.

We also want to know that the client has some level of support, meaning relationships, skills, or effective ways of taking care of themselves when needed.

In EMDR processing, the *timing and setting* are crucial and must be tailored to each client's unique needs. Adjustments may be necessary for shorter sessions or based on the complexity of the issues being addressed. When working remotely, practitioners should assess clients' safety and privacy in their home (virtual) environments, determining whether to engage in deeper processing or to focus on smaller targets. Similarly, in school settings or under insurance constraints, the available session length can dictate the depth of processing that is feasible.

A client's willingness to engage with past concerns is essential for effective outcomes. The clinician maintains control over bilateral stimulation, whether through eye movements or other methods, while guiding the client's participation in a balanced and effective manner.

For those utilizing technology, various apps and devices offer effective means for BLS but require consistent monitoring of client responses. Telehealth practitioners must also adapt their techniques accordingly, especially for clients who may experience discomfort with specific forms of stimulation.

Overall, *clear communication*, *proper pacing*, and *accommodating individual client needs* are key factors for successful EMDR sessions. And this is only accomplished by attuning to the client's needs and presentation.

Titrated Attuned Processing

There are levels of processing that can be worked with, depending on the client's ability to stay in the room with the clinician. EMDR, as described by Shapiro, is full-on processing of the entire neurological network using bilateral stimulation at what can be called "full speed." This looks like thirty laps or more of BLS at a fast pace—as fast as the client can manage. Again, this stirs up the entire negative neural network, and the mind does the job of processing and clearing the feelings associated with the thoughts of the events.

With attuned precision, we can determine whether to use full-on EMDR or, if needed, cut the laps down so the mind can work more easily with less input from the brain. This might be considered somewhat restricted processing. Finally, we can slow it down further using what Shapiro called EMD: only 10 to 13 laps of processing at a fast speed, focusing on one event (target) at a time. Think of this like a buffet—a buffet of trauma trails in the system. EMD lets us process one bite at a time instead of the whole buffet of trauma memory.

Our attunement to the client determines the best way to proceed. Keep in mind that the client does not know what we are calibrating, so we can slow down or speed up at will. When we see that the client can handle more, we can move into longer sets, but we know that, if needed, we can step back down.

Processing Interventions

Regarding the AIP approach to therapy during processing, the client's adaptive processing system consolidates networks. What this means is we have a negative neurological network that harbors trauma information. When we process—because we have worked with the adaptive network to consolidate the negative into the positive—the client experiences relief.

Occasionally, the flow of information and consolidation is disrupted, leading to stalled processing. It is the clinician's task to keep the processing moving, and as clinicians, we have to be attuned to what is disrupting the processing.

We need to provide the least invasive and intrusive intervention to reactivate the processing. This would also minimize clinical interruptions to the client's own AIP process.

We will examine several interventions that can aid in resolving stalled processing. We could change the bilateral stimulus. In many situations, when processing stops, changing either the speed, direction, or type of bilateral stimulus is all that's needed to resume processing.

We could, for example, if we're using eye movements, change from horizontal to diagonal. Or we could change the rhythm of the tapping. We could, if we're changing the rhythm of tapping, change the speed, the tension, or any other way of doing that. We could tap twice on one knee, once on the other knee—whatever seems to be a way to make it work. The objective here is to get out of a rhythm and into a different rhythm, which will jolt the processing to start up again.

Now, when a client is looping—meaning the client goes back to the same idea and the same response, time after time, reporting the same images, thoughts, or sensations—one way to change this is to ask: *"What are you noticing now?"* or *"What are you thinking?"* or *"How is it for you?"* You could also ask the client, *"What do you notice in your body?"*—and then go with that.

If a client is fixated, we could change the focus of the incident. For example, if a client had been attacked by somebody and was fixated on the face, arm, or hand of the perpetrator, we could ask them to focus on what the perpetrator said or on something else in the environment of the incident.

The next thing to consider is secondary gains. If the client feels (knowingly or unknowingly) that processing is attempting to change something that may not be in their best interest, real or perceived, the client might experience what we call a secondary gain. Taking those words apart—*secondary gain*—means that the client has something to gain by holding on to the difficulty and the behaviors that create the maladaptive–adaptive response.

A good example of this would be, say, you're working with a veteran, and if they healed, then their money—their benefits—would be taken away. Therefore, their internal system has a vested interest in staying ill.

Now, it might be necessary, with secondary gains, to stop for a moment and provide alternative strategies or new learnings. It may also be important to advise the client that your note-taking will not reveal anything that would be harmful to them.

Another thing to consider is whether there are incongruent structures in their negative and positive beliefs. For example, if an adaptive belief is externally focused, then chances are the client will not be able to process successfully. An example of this would be if the negative belief is *"I am unimportant,"* and the adaptive or positive belief is *"I am important,"* but the importance depends on someone else providing information about themselves. That is not actually a positive belief. It is a belief that someone is doing something for them, which will not strengthen them if they must rely on others. So, we have to look at that.

The AIP system cannot process other people's behaviors or beliefs. If we identify an adaptive belief as externally focused, then we must reframe it to have an internal locus. For instance, if the negative belief is *"I'm unimportant,"* then the client could say to themselves, *"I have value and self-worth, regardless."*

Let's look at the word *regardless.* The word "regardless" removes externals from the scenario and allows the unconscious mind to determine the positive belief simply because it is about the client, not about anybody else doing something for them.

The positive belief might be unrealistic. So, for example, if you have a perpetrator on a child, and the child has felt a sense of powerlessness, a child can never be adaptive to *"I am powerful"* because a child cannot be powerful in that sort of situation.

However, a choice, potentially, something to look at would be *"I can control what I can, regardless of whether I am good or not."*

Now, there may be some underlying blocking beliefs, such as fears that are preventing proper processing. For example, a negative belief is that *"I am unsafe when I express feelings."* An adaptive thought could be, *"I can begin to learn how to express feelings,"* or another thought would be, *"I can express feelings regardless."*

Now, in addition to what we've already mentioned, Francine Shapiro, in her book, describes something called cognitive interweaving. Cognitive interweaves are essentially questions that we ask the client, which are not meant to be answered externally.

This means that we are challenging the unconscious mind to hear a question that will reveal a truth the client either cognitively or experientially does not perceive. The unconscious mind is actually challenged by a more powerful truth that makes sense and works towards being noticed.

When processing memories, breakdowns in the flow of information may occur, necessitating the interweaving of memories.

Breaking a fight-or-flight-freeze response, knowing that life goes on, and updating to the present could be necessary. And if that's the case, you might say something like, *"It's over, it's in the past, you're here now,"* and go with that.

Another possibility—if one has a childhood memory that does not have adaptive information to resolve a situation, while processing a childhood abuse memory, and the child still feels it's their fault, you could say something like: *"I'm confused. If a child that you know were being hurt like that, would it be their fault?"* Now, when we ask those sorts of questions and do not expect or wait for an answer, you can only imagine that the unconscious mind answers them and updates the system with real information that is useful and adaptive.

So, the purpose of the interweave is to reestablish the linkage between the known adaptive network and the negative network, thereby reactivating the processing. Now, these interweaves are not to be discussed, and you want to trust your clinical instinct and attunement to the client's needs.

Now, if you've done a good, thorough biopsychosocial in the beginning, you're going to understand their history, beliefs, and cognitions. You also need to understand the client's developmental stage at the time the trauma occurred.

If you think you might need a cognitive interweave, consider doing one more set of bilateral exercises to see if the interweave is still necessary. And then you can just ask the question, and then just say, *"Go with that"* rather than *"Let's talk about that."*

When we're doing cognitive interweaves, we will not talk about it; we will simply allow the mind to process the new information.

The next consideration is managing the processing within the window of tolerance. We know that optimal processing occurs when the client is halfway in the experience and halfway in the present—in your office or online.

The client maintains that dual awareness: one foot in the present, one foot in the past. They are aware of their present orientation, responsiveness, and ability to manage and tolerate stress.

If they're over-accessing their trauma memories, they may become hypo-aroused. They might be shut down, numb, frozen, or withdrawn. Or they may become hyper-aroused, acting out, hypervigilant, or anxious.

And if they're under-accessing, the client may be too much in the present and does not feel the emotional charge of the incident required for processing. If they're over-accessing, we can pendulate. Pendulation means we ask the client to notice elements in the room that draw their attention to the present time, not the time of trauma.

We can restrict the bilateral stimulus by using fewer saccades or fewer laps. We can also contain by working with shorter, smaller targets. If they're under-accessing, we might adjust the bilateral and shift focus to the body. And if they're in the optimal processing window, we proceed with standard EMDR.

This brings us to managing higher levels of emotion during processing, while still staying within that optimal window. What we learn is that we can titrate the bilateral stimulus.

The more laps we do, the more stimulus is applied to the negative neural network, and the more emotions and sensations may surface. If we're approaching the upper edge of the window of tolerance, we can simply slow it down by doing fewer laps of bilateral.

It's not unusual to experience increased emotional intensity during EMDR. In fact, things often intensify before they release.

This does not mean the client is being re-traumatized. Instead, the client is observing the memory, not reliving it. The bilateral stimulus helps release and integrate that memory into the adaptive network.

We can support the client through this process by gently saying things like:

It's over now.

You're here with me.

It happened a long time ago.

It's in the past.

You're safe now.

Watch it like you're watching scenery from a car window.

And above all, ensure you and the client have previously agreed on a stop signal—a clear, nonverbal cue. If the client uses it, you stop immediately. Respect for that signal is non-negotiable.

During processing, we can instruct the client to take a deep breath and even assist them with breathing—this models attunement and connection. Breathe with the client. Say, *"Take a deep breath. Let it go. Now return to the target memory" (or return to what you are noticing now).*

When we wish to restrict processing, we reduce the bilateral to 10–15 seconds, then prompt a breath and ask, *"How disturbing is it now? On a scale from 0 to 10, where 0 means no disturbance and 10 is the highest you can imagine?"*

If the client continues to exceed their window of tolerance, remaining either hyper- or hypo-aroused, and restricted sets aren't effective, then transition to pendulation or fragment the target, and sometimes both.

To pendulate, at the end of each restricted set, ask them to name five things they can see in the room. Then, there are four things they can hear. This is grounding using the 5-4-3-2-1 technique you taught them earlier during Phase Two of EMDR (preparation).

You'll go back and forth from processing to grounding—step by step, a little at a time.

If needed, fragment the target. Take only a small part of the memory, not the most disturbing part. For instance, when thinking about a perpetrator, start with just the face. Ask, *"How disturbing is that now?"* Then shift to just the arms that were hitting: *"How disturbing is that now?"* This allows for manageable entry points into the trauma without overwhelming the system.

Take it a little at a time. We can transition through processing states, from standard to contained, from contained to restricted, and then back to standard, as needed. We don't always have to explain this to the client or ask them what to do. A useful metaphor here is driving on black ice for those of us who live in or are familiar with winter conditions. When we hit black ice, we don't slam on the brakes, and we don't step on the gas—we let the car decelerate naturally. The same applies in EMDR processing: transitioning from standard processing to contained or restricted processing is about adjusting the pace to match what the client's system can tolerate. It's about knowing how fast we can safely go and how skillfully we can steer the EMDR car without losing control.

And this is all part of attuning to the client.

Cultivating Flexibility, Rhythm, and Clinical Judgment

Legal Considerations

When clients are involved in legal cases, particularly those related to traumatic assault, abuse, or theft, timing is everything. EMDR is highly effective at reducing the emotional intensity of traumatic memories, which can alter the emotional presentation of a client's testimony. If a client appears emotionally neutral or detached while testifying, it may unintentionally undermine the gravity of their experience in the eyes of the court. For this reason, it may be wise to encourage the client to consult their attorney before proceeding with reprocessing the target trauma.

However, EMDR can still be useful in preparation for legal proceedings. We can work on processing the anticipated courtroom experience, including targets such as facing the perpetrator, being cross-examined, or sitting in the courtroom. These anticipatory triggers are often charged with fear and anxiety and can be addressed while preserving the emotional tone of the original traumatic memory.

Still, it's essential to remember that EMDR can lead to new insights, emotions, and sensations. These shifts may emerge spontaneously and could have implications in a legal setting. So, with the client's consent, clinicians may need to communicate with their lawyer. The decision to process the event itself or to focus solely on the legal context must be made collaboratively and carefully, with clinical attunement and ethical responsibility at the forefront.

Understanding Self-Harm and Suicide

Self-harm is often a coping mechanism—a protective adaptation used by clients who are unable to regulate their internal emotional states. When a client externalizes pain through cutting, burning, or other forms of harm, it typically signals that they're not yet resourced enough to handle the emotional activation that full EMDR processing can trigger.

In these cases, we must slow down. More grounding. More resourcing. More containment.

Instead of full EMDR, we might work with EMD—fewer laps of bilateral stimulation—and smaller targets. Think of it like this: the client doesn't need to chew the entire trauma at once. We're just asking them to take a bite, to engage with a tiny, manageable segment of their distress, not the whole thing in one overwhelming swoop.

For example, rather than processing the entirety of an assault, we might focus only on the sound of footsteps, or the feeling of cold air, or the moment the door opened: tiny pieces, one at a time.

Dual Awareness and Affect Regulation

A central goal in EMDR therapy is to help clients maintain dual awareness—the ability to maintain a balance between the past and the present. When this is achieved, the client can engage the traumatic memory without becoming dysregulated. This doesn't mean they won't feel—instead, it means they'll feel without flooding or shutting down.

Clients should be able to move between positive and negative affective states, returning to the present moment with relative ease. If we suspect dissociation, we can use tools like the Dissociative Experiences Scale (DES), the Adverse Childhood Experiences (ACEs) questionnaire, or the MID-60 to assess their vulnerability.

If scores are elevated, emphasize grounding techniques, teach containment, and ensure they have enough internal scaffolding to return to the present if they begin to drift or dissociate. In cases of highly dissociated clients, we would have to work longer and more intensely in the preparation phase. In addition, consider taking more in-depth training in using EMDR therapy with dissociated clients.

Support Systems

It is vital to ascertain whether clients have a support network, such as friends or family. For clients who are agoraphobic or isolated, helping them build or rebuild relationships becomes essential. If clinician contact becomes necessary outside of the session, identifying a reliable support person is crucial—someone who can assist the client in case of emergencies or emotional crises.

The desensitization phase of EMDR is pivotal for helping clients process and reduce the emotional distress linked to traumatic memories. Through bilateral stimulation, which may involve eye movements, tapping, or auditory tones, clients gradually work to lower the emotional charge associated with trauma while maintaining dual awareness: one foot in the present, the other in the past.

This phase demands careful preparation, client-specific tailoring, and emotional attunement. Not all individuals are ready for full EMDR processing, which engages the entire neurological network. Some clients may require restricted or contained processing depending on their stabilization level and risk factors, such as suicidality, dissociation, or self-harming tendencies.

Clinicians must ensure that clients have established grounding skills, affect regulation, and can remain within their window of tolerance. Throughout processing, it's essential to monitor their feedback using tools like the SUD scale, which helps determine whether to continue, pause, or adjust the BLS protocol.

Medical conditions, environmental safety, and specific psychosocial dynamics also influence the success of EMDR. For example, clients with epilepsy, migraines, TBI, or visual sensitivities may need non-visual BLS methods. Similarly, clients in remote settings or those subject to legal constraints may require adjustments in timing and content.

Throughout the desensitization phase, clinicians must stay attuned to the client's nonverbal cues, such as changes in posture, breath, vocal tone, or subtle physical reactions. These signals often reveal internal responses before words do. In cases of disruption or stalled processing, cognitive interweaves may be used to stimulate the AIP system. These interweaves are non-intrusive questions that challenge maladaptive beliefs by engaging the client's unconscious mind to explore more adaptive truths.

Whether navigating legal considerations, helping clients with histories of self-harm, or ensuring a stable external support system, EMDR requires clinicians to approach therapy with flexibility, compassion, and clinical precision. The effectiveness of desensitization rests not only in the technique itself, but in the clinician's empathic connection, clear communication, and ability to adapt to each client's unique emotional terrain.

Phase 5—Attunement and Installation in EMDR Therapy

In this next phase of EMDR, we shift our focus to installation, where we work with the positive cognition identified during the earlier stages of treatment. It is essential to understand that the EMDR process is fluid, and as clients move through their memories, this positive belief may evolve, deepen, or even change entirely.

Shifting from Maladaptive to Adaptive Cognition

As clients reprocess their traumatic experiences, new adaptive insights often emerge. Initially, clients may meet painful memories through the lens of maladaptive beliefs formed during traumatic events—beliefs rooted in survival rather than authentic self-understanding.

Over time, however, these survival-based beliefs and coping strategies, once necessary, can become maladaptive in the present. The purpose of this phase is to support a conscious and neurological shift from old, limiting beliefs toward a more adaptive internal framework.

As processing unfolds and disturbing emotions are desensitized, the client's positive belief becomes more than just a statement—it begins to take root neurologically. The adaptive network strengthens, allowing for a deeper conviction and a clearer sense of self.

In some cases, the original positive cognition may require adjustment as new insights surface. The belief *"I can handle it"* might evolve into *"I am strong and safe now, regardless."* The client's core narrative begins to shift, replacing trauma-informed self-concepts with empowered, resilient, and grounded truths.

Evaluating the Positive Cognition

To gauge the current suitability of the positive cognition, clinicians can ask the following question: *"When you think of the original incident, does the positive cognition still fit, or could there be a better one?"* The focus here is on ensuring that the belief remains an internal one—an *"I am"* statement that defines the client without requiring external validation.

Once the client affirms an internal locus of control in their positive cognition, we can proceed to enhance its validity. This is referred to as the Validity of Cognition (VOC). To do this, clients are instructed to hold the original incident and the positive cognition simultaneously while rating how true the cognition feels (or is) on a scale of 1 to 7 (1 being "totally false" and 7 being "totally true").

Strengthening the Positive Cognition

To reinforce the positive cognition, clinicians guide clients through a series of bilateral stimulus sets at a processing speed for approximately 10 to 15 seconds (around 12 sweeps). After this, clinicians will reassess the VOC: *"When you think of the incident and your positive cognition, how true does it feel now?"* The process of strengthening continues until the VOC reaches a score of 7 or until no further increase is noted.

Attunement and Signs of Release

In this phase, attunement is focused on observing the client's emotional and physical release. This may manifest as changes in breathing patterns, facial expressions, or smiles. Sometimes, clients may experience tears, and it's essential to check whether these are tears of joy or another emotional release.

Clinicians must pay attention to nonverbal cues, such as shoulder movement, breathing, hand tension, and leg tension, among others, which indicate progress and restoration of strength within the client's system.

In the installation phase of EMDR therapy, our focus shifts to reinforcing the client's positive cognitions that have emerged through processing. The goal is to solidify and enhance their sense of self and their ability to navigate life's challenges. We begin by assessing the initial positive belief, recognizing that processing often leads to a refined and strengthened internal narrative, which in turn leads to an adaptive belief about oneself.

As clients integrate these experiences, they may discover that their previously maladaptive-adaptive behaviors are shifting toward truly adaptive responses. We then assess the client's internal locus of control by having the client report how they feel and whether the positive cognition still resonates with them.

To solidify this, we assess the Validity of Cognition, the VOC, using a scale of 1 to 7, and strengthen it through bilateral stimulation of processing speed until a sense of being grounded is achieved, paving the way for Phase 6 and beyond. Throughout this process, attunement is paramount; we remain vigilant in observing and responding to physical cues, reading the body's response to assess and support the client as they experience release, healing, and the restoration of strength within their system.

Phase 6—Attunement and Body Scan in EMDR Therapy

Phase 6 of EMDR therapy, aptly referred to as the body scan, shifts the focus to processing any lingering physical sensations that may persist after the psychological work has been completed. As Bessel van der Kolk famously stated, *"The Body Keeps the Score,"* underscoring the profound connection between trauma and bodily sensations. When we address trauma therapeutically, it is crucial to recognize that the body often retains echoes of those traumatic experiences, even after cognitive processing appears to be complete.

During the body scan phase, our role is to assist clients in identifying and processing these somatic remnants. We guide them by prompting them to think of the original incident alongside their positive cognition, encouraging them to perform a thorough head-to-toe scan of their bodies. As they do this, we invite them to report any sensations they experience, which may reflect their earlier processing work.

An attentive therapist remains acutely aware of the client's physical cues and behaviors throughout this process. For example, observing where clients place their hands can provide insights into their internal states. A client holding their hands on their stomach or upper chest may be signaling areas of anxiety or discomfort. Or sometimes a client will clench their throat. This level of attunement not only facilitates better communication but also enhances the therapist's ability to respond effectively to the client's needs.

The goal of the body scan is to identify any residual physiological responses stemming from the traumatic experience. Once a client identifies specific sensations, the therapist encourages them to stay attuned to these feelings, helping them focus on any existing discomfort or tension. If sensations are detected, we employ bilateral stimulation—approximately 10 to 15 seconds, or 11 to 12 sets of stimulation at a processing speed—to facilitate the release of these feelings. The process continues until clients report a state of calm, neutrality, or sometimes sensations of lightness or tingling.

It's important to note that positive sensations are indicators of progress. Once a client reports a shift toward calmness, we may perform one additional round of bilateral stimulation before transitioning to Phase 7, which centers on closure.

In the body scan stage of EMDR therapy, it is essential to acknowledge the importance of processing any residual physical sensations associated with trauma. By integrating the principles of attunement, therapists can effectively guide clients in identifying and addressing these somatic remnants, ultimately facilitating a deeper healing experience. As clients engage in a thorough body scan, observing their physical responses helps them reconnect with their bodies while utilizing bilateral stimulation to promote stability and calm. This phase not only reinforces the therapeutic work already completed but also sets the stage for a gentle transition into closure, marking another step in the journey toward holistic healing and integration.

Keeping in mind, during the body scan, we aim to identify the somatic remnants of the processing. We may prompt clients to think of the original incident and their positive cognition while scanning their bodies for sensations. Any sensations reported could be directly related to the processing work. It is vital for clients to focus on these body sensations while the therapist attentively observes their physical responses, taking note of where they place their hands, for instance, as this can indicate areas of anxiety.

While the body scan aims to identify leftover physiological responses from trauma, it is worth noting that clients may sometimes report sensations unrelated to the trauma. For instance, a client might feel stomach discomfort that is simply hunger rather than a reflection of trauma. Additionally, actual physical pain or discomfort due to medical reasons should be recognized, and therapists should not expect those sensations to be processed until a pain protocol is used for some relief. And note that if there is a physical (medical) issue, EMDR may not resolve it, but it may help the client manage it.

It is possible that conducting a body scan, which involves checking the client's body from head to toe for any disturbances, could be reflective of unfinished targets or events in the neurological network that are begging to be processed. It's kind of like dormant memories that want to be healed, as the memories the client worked on are resolved.

In addition, it is also possible that a client is not accustomed to resolution, so it's a good idea to take the time with the client, noticing the absence of angst as it is reflected in both the body and mind. If, by chance, there is no absolute recognition that the target was worked on in the session, meaning the work is incomplete, we can contain it by placing the image, feeling, or representation in a container and agreeing to work with it in a future session. If there are many targets, it is not uncommon for the body to signal that there is more work to be done.

Phases 7–8: Closure and Re-evaluation with Compassion

A completed session might look like this: the SUD is zero, the VOC is seven, and the body scan is neutral. In Phase 7, closure, we simply want to debrief. We can discuss the processing experience, including insights and realizations, and how the process is affecting the client.

How do we work with this? Pretty simple—we ask the client what they notice. We ask them to reflect on what has changed and how they know it has changed. Keeping attuned to the client, it's important to remember that each individual has their own way of reporting change. Some will express a cognitive understanding, others will report somatic differences, and some might just say something like, *"It's blank inside,"* where it was cluttered before processing.

It is in the closure phase that we also gather information for a possible next session. What we are listening for are comments and musings about what might still be lingering in the neurological network—anything that remains outstanding. Remember that when we process neurologically, we're often working through interconnected things. Each target may not be a standalone. Hebb's axiom applies here: things that are wired together fire together, which also implies that things that are wired together process together.

It is also during closure that we can detect or observe the underpinnings of aspects of self that are protecting the client from letting go of angst for the sake of protection. It's important to note these observations for the next session.

This discussion actually helps consolidate the network. Network consolidation means that the client begins to clearly understand what has happened—that something within them has shifted—and they no longer experience the extreme feelings or sensations tied to the traumatic event(s). They likely will, however, remember that the event happened.

In closing, we always want to remind the client that processing will continue. They may experience thoughts, feelings, dreams, or physical sensations after leaving the session. If it's appropriate, the clinician can suggest ways for the client to track this ongoing processing. For example, the clinician might say: "I welcome you to write down any thoughts or feelings that come up after this session. If anything feels particularly sticky, I'd like to hear about it when we meet again. These details help guide us in determining the next steps in processing your trauma."

We also advise every clinician to complete summary notes once the session is finished. It's essential to document where the target began—whether it was in the past, present, or future. Note how the processing was conducted: Was it standard EMDR? Was it contained or restricted EMD?

Record what was targeted: the negative belief, the positive belief, the VOC, the emotions associated with it, the SUD score, and the body location. After the session, post-session information should be added, including the outcome—what was the SUD? What was the VOC?

Additionally, note whether stabilization was required—such as grounding, containment, or any other methods. Include a few treatment notes, and if you deem it appropriate, outline any further treatment recommendations or directions for the next session.

Now, a question comes up: what do we do if there's unfinished processing—if the SUD is greater than zero?

If you're doing EMDR with unrestricted processing, it's normal and somewhat expected that some targets may require more than one session to complete. This is not a failure of the process—it's simply the nature of deep, layered trauma work.

As you approach the end of your session and notice that the SUD has not come down significantly—or has not reached zero, or what you may deem as ecological closure—you can gently inform the client that you're nearing the end of your time together. Offering the client agency, you might ask, *"Would you like to do one more set or stop here for today?"* From there, proceed to stabilize as needed.

Ground and stabilize the client using the techniques already established earlier in your work. By this point, you should know which stabilization strategies are most effective for the client and which are not. Go with what you know works. If necessary, use the client's containment strategy to hold what remains unfinished.

Then, debrief by asking the client what they've learned from the session. After that, close with care and clarity.

A related question often arises: What does "ecological SUD" mean?

When we talk about ecological SUD, we're acknowledging that some clients may need to retain a manageable level of alertness or disturbance for safety-related reasons. For instance, first responders may need to stay somewhat hypervigilant due to the demands of their roles. Their SUD might not reach zero, and that's okay, as long as it's not overwhelming.

Another example might be clients with medical conditions who must stay vigilant about symptoms or health concerns. In such cases, the goal isn't necessarily full resolution, but manageable integration.

This kind of work can also be a time of powerful self-discovery. Clients may experience a spontaneous shift in their positive beliefs. As trauma is cleared, a deeper, more authentic belief about the self may emerge—one that has been buried under years of coping and adaptation. When this happens, adopt the new, positive cognition. Allow it to "morph" into a more relevant, meaningful version. If so, return to the installation phase and, if appropriate, proceed to future templates to reinforce the client's newfound strength and resilience.

Phase 8—Attunement and Re-Evaluation

Phase 8 is re-evaluation, which begins when the client returns to the office (or virtual) after their last EMDR (or other) session.

Begin by asking the client what they have been experiencing since the last session. This should be an open-ended, gently vague question—something like, *"When you think about what we worked on last time, what are you experiencing now?"* The client's response will reveal whether the target or issue addressed previously has been resolved or still requires attention, or whether other issues in their neural network have emerged.

Once you have that information, determine the current SUD. If necessary, you can return directly to reprocessing to bring the SUD to a zero or to a level that is ecologically relevant and sustainable for the client.

Remember, most importantly, ecological relevance refers to the reality that some clients may need to retain a small amount of disturbance or a felt sense of the issue for reasons of perceived or actual safety. For them, a complete absence of disturbance might feel unsafe. In these situations, attunement is key—allow the client to define what "resolved enough" feels like.

The idea is to ensure that when we are processing and desensitizing a "target," the target is actually in the past. An ecological remnant of disturbance may be significant for the client to retain. A good example of this can be seen in the roles of first responders, including police officers, firefighters, EMTs, doctors, nurses, teachers, and even therapists. If individuals who regularly respond to danger lose their sense of hypervigilance, they may put themselves at risk.

In light of how the past informs the present, retaining a modicum of disturbance may be essential for specific clients. The key question is: Does this residual disturbance hamper or impede the client's life and well-being? If it does, we would want to continue processing the target event until the client can report that the memory no longer interferes with their life in meaningful or consequential ways.

Why Some Clients Hesitate to Continue EMDR Therapy After Initial Success

It's a question that often arises and is entirely understandable. Have you ever had a client completely resolve a significant memory during an EMDR session, only to return the following week and say, *"Hey, can we just talk today?"*

What's going on? After weeks or months of preparation and the successful clearing of a painful memory, why wouldn't they want to continue EMDR right away?

Let's explore a few scenarios. The recommendations for moving forward will depend on which situation applies.

Scenario 1: A Positive Experience with EMDR

First, let's consider clients who had a successful EMDR session—no major disruptions, no difficult after-effects—and felt that the memory had been fully resolved. They may even be surprised by how well the process worked. So why hesitate?

Clients can learn multiple things simultaneously. On the one hand, they discover that healing can occur quickly and deeply. That realization is both empowering and comforting. On the other hand, they may also learn that EMDR can be intense, physically and emotionally exhausting in ways they didn't expect or can't always control.

Some clients may arrive at their next session after a rough week, poor sleep, or with life plans that could be disrupted by emotional processing. They weigh the benefits of working with you—feeling safe and supported—against the unpredictable nature of trauma work.

In these cases, it's vital to have an open and compassionate conversation. Asking, *"What makes you feel hesitant about continuing EMDR right now?"* can reveal underlying concerns and guide your next steps. It's also essential to honor the client's flow. If needed, help them contain any remaining thoughts, emotions, or body sensations for future work. Timing matters. It could be possible that avoidance is at play. In that case, targeting avoidance, saying, *"Just how much do you want to not go further with processing?"* Take a SUD, process it using BLS for about 10-12 laps, and continue until the SUD stops changing. Then we ask if the client would like to proceed with their target sequence plan.

Scenario 2: Difficulties During or After Sessions

In another scenario, a client may have had a difficult session. The emotions were overwhelming, and they faced issues they were hoping to avoid. When this happens, it can feel disorienting—not just to the client but also to the therapist.

However, such experiences are not failures. They are feedback. They present valuable opportunities for reflection, learning, and growth. A challenging EMDR session can reveal hidden resistances, unprocessed layers, or maladaptive coping strategies that are ripe for transformation and change. When approached with care and curiosity, these moments can strengthen the therapeutic alliance and pave the way for more effective work moving forward.

Clients may not always understand what options exist for managing their distress. If they experience a challenging session, we can reassure them that it's okay—we don't have to return to that same material right away. We can pivot to more manageable memories, reinforce their coping strategies, or teach them how to approach their emotions gradually.

Guidance from resources such as *EMDR with Complex Trauma* by Thomas Zimmerman can offer helpful strategies for clients who need additional support. It's crucial to ask clients about their difficulties. Even if they don't fully understand their options, they can usually articulate what they're feeling or experiencing.

Scenario 3: Addressing Lower Levels of Distress

A common dilemma arises when a client processes a memory from an SUD rating of 8 down to 2 in a single session. In the following session, they might say that 2 is "good enough" and show little interest in revisiting it. From their point of view, it makes sense—a SUD of 2 doesn't feel intrusive, and they may have more pressing concerns in the present.

In these cases, it's important to approach their reluctance collaboratively. Help clients understand that fully resolving the memory can free up emotional and cognitive bandwidth, making it easier to manage future challenges. Reassure them that clearing out lingering residue can yield meaningful long-term benefits. However, always express empathy for their present focus and avoid applying pressure. Trust and pacing are crucial.

General Suggestions for Addressing Client Hesitations

Encourage open and honest dialogue about any hesitations your clients may have. Approach these conversations without an agenda. Follow their lead, but if a clinical dilemma arises, share that dilemma with them. Their feedback can provide valuable insights and guide your next steps.

If the SUD remains above zero at the end of a session, it's essential to ground the client. Use techniques such as guided imagery, visualizing a peaceful place, or containment exercises to stabilize them. This helps them feel safe between sessions and supports emotional regulation.

Continuing the Process

Please note that EMDR processing may require multiple sessions. Each session should ideally conclude with a moment of reflection to help consolidate what's been learned and reinforce the neural connections formed during the work.

Update your treatment notes template as needed to accurately reflect session details. Good documentation not only serves as a clinical roadmap but also functions as a legal safeguard. Include information such as the client's presenting concerns, session number, specific target addressed, and outcome (e.g., SUD, VOC, body location).

Specific populations—such as first responders or those facing ongoing trauma—may not reach a zero SUD for ecological reasons. In these cases, blend work on past events with resource-building strategies to prepare them for future challenges. Helping these clients manage hypervigilance while preserving functionality is often the therapeutic goal.

Cognitive Interweaves During Processing

For those familiar with Ericksonian language patterns (from Milton Erickson), we understand the power of the unconscious mind in trauma resolution.

To keep the client supported during processing, you can use gentle, indirect phrases such as:

- *"You can nurture yourself through this experience."*
- *"Notice what that might be like for you."*

To emphasize safety and orientation, say:

- *"It's over. You're here now."*
- *"This happened in the past, and you're in my office now."*

These suggestions aren't prompts for verbal replies. We're speaking to the unconscious mind, which does the deeper work. These phrases gently guide the client's awareness without demanding cognitive effort.

To help with distancing, use metaphors:

- Think of it like scenery passing by from a car or on your iPad.
- In a video by clinician Bob Tinker, he uses the metaphor of a train. Clients are encouraged to imagine themselves on the

train, looking out the window as the scenery—memories and emotions—pass by.

These tools support clients as they move through the discomfort of processing, reminding them of safety, grounding them in the present, and helping them gently distance themselves from the intensity of past experiences.

Always remind clients of their stop signal and respect their need to pause when they request it. Let them know it's perfectly okay to take a break and recharge if necessary. Honoring their choices and boundaries strengthens trust and reinforces their sense of safety and agency in the therapeutic space.

Managing Processing and the Window of Tolerance

Effectively managing a client's processing requires staying within their window of tolerance. When clients become hyper-aroused, they may experience overwhelming emotions and physical sensations, potentially reliving the trauma. This can trigger fight, flight, freeze, or fawn responses, which are usually driven by terror rather than ordinary fear.

On the other end of the spectrum, hypo-arousal can lead to emotional shutdown, numbness, dissociation, or a marked lack of responsiveness. Hyper-arousal often manifests as externalized behaviors—such as tension, rapid speech, and restlessness—while hypo-arousal is more internalized, presenting as disconnection, flat affect, or sluggish movements.

Both states signal that the client is outside their capacity to cope with internal stimuli and may begin to rely on adaptive—but ultimately maladaptive—coping strategies.

Interventions When Exceeding Tolerance

If a client exceeds their window of tolerance during processing, slow down the pace. Offer a gentle, running verbal narrative of what's happening. Though it may seem counterintuitive, talking more during these moments can help bring the client back to the present.

As you engage in bilateral stimulation, encourage the client to simply notice what is happening internally, without expecting verbal responses. This allows the unconscious mind to engage, to uncover adaptive truths, and promote internal balance.

Help ground the client in time and place. Remind them:

- *"You're here in my office now."*
- *"What we're processing is from the past."*

To support geographical orientation and distancing, encourage visualizations—watching the memory pass by like scenery from a moving vehicle, such as a car, train, or iPad.

Techniques for Processing

To regulate emotional intensity, shorten the duration of bilateral stimulation by limiting sets to 10 or 15 seconds when necessary. At the end of each set, give clear and calming directions:

- *"Take a few deep breaths."*
- *"Notice how your body feels right now."*

Modeling this yourself by syncing your breath with theirs can enhance attunement.

After each set, invite the client to return to the target memory by asking something like:

- *"What do you notice now when you think of where we started?"*

This incremental checking-in approach helps the client stay within their window of tolerance and provides a rhythm to the work that supports emotional containment.

Clinical Judgment is Key

EMDR is not a rigid protocol; it requires ongoing attunement and adaptation to individual needs. While knowledge of the phases and techniques is essential, attunement to the client's moment-to-moment experience is critical. We must learn the basic protocol in order to adapt it for the client's well-being.

If dysregulation arises:

- Shorten the stimulation sets.
- Limit the duration to fewer seconds.
- Integrate grounding strategies, such as slow breathing, naming objects in the room, or focusing on the present moment.

Continuously monitor their SUD level throughout the session and adjust accordingly.

This responsive, client-centric approach allows for safe and effective trauma processing while supporting the client's overall sense of agency and stability.

Advanced Techniques

If a client remains in a state of hypo-arousal or hyper-arousal despite attempts to regulate, it may be time to transition techniques. One effective method is pendulation, which involves alternating between the traumatic material and grounding resources. This is similar to the 5-4-3-2-1 grounding exercise and helps re-anchor the client in the present while still allowing for gradual processing of the traumatic memory.

Another option is fragmenting the target—breaking down the trauma into manageable pieces. Rather than asking the client to focus on the entire traumatic event or the worst part of the event, you might guide them to focus on a single detail, such as the sound of a door closing or the expression on the perpetrator's face. This reduces the emotional intensity and gives the client more control. (Dolores Mosquera, Tip of the Finger Processing). Step by step, you can process a whole event.

Using Titration Techniques

The titration technique allows for flexible, client-responsive processing. You adjust the speed, intensity, and duration of bilateral stimulation based on how the client is responding moment to moment. Think of it metaphorically: you're driving the EMDR car, and the client is sitting in the front seat with you. They're telling you where they want to go, and you're adjusting the route and speed accordingly.

To slow down processing, reduce the number of laps per set, or shorten the stimulation duration. To accelerate, increase the number of laps. It's about constant calibration and attunement, carefully watching for signs of overwhelm or disengagement.

Addressing Client Concerns and Fears

If a client expresses hesitation or fear about processing, acknowledge and explore it with compassion. Use a 0–10 scale to assess their level of avoidance (from Jim Knipe, EMDR Toolbox):

- *"How much would you say you want to avoid this right now, on a scale of zero to ten?"*

This helps quantify their resistance and opens the door to deeper conversations. Reassure them that processing does not diminish their strength or take away their ability to function in future challenges. If their SUD increases when thinking about the trauma, consider doing a CID to reduce avoidance and help them re-engage with the work safely.

If a core belief emerges—such as *"It's not safe to feel"*—this can become a new target in itself. Explore the origins of that belief and strive to develop a more adaptive, reality-based cognition that supports healing and growth.

Reviewing Progress in Follow-up Sessions

During the re-evaluation phase (Phase 8), begin with a global check-in:

- *"How has your week been since our last session?"*

This broad question allows the client to lead the conversation and share what feels most important without forcing them to provide unnecessary details.

From there, assess how the previously targeted material has settled. Check the current SUD level for that target. If it remains above zero, continue processing. If the client seems ready, introduce the next target with clarity and structure, especially if the next issue relates to anxiety, avoidance, or anticipatory distress.

General Suggestions for Addressing Client Hesitations

Create an open and non-judgmental space where clients can express their hesitations freely. Approach these conversations without a fixed agenda. When resistance becomes a clinical dilemma, bring it to the client's attention with transparency and clarity. Let them be part of the decision-making process.

Their feedback isn't just helpful; it's necessary. It will guide the pacing, direction, and depth of your work together, ensuring the process remains safe, collaborative, and transformative.

Dissociation: What to Do if a Client Gets Stuck

When working with EMDR therapy, we understand that processing occurs in the present moment, and what is processed is registered through the client's neurological system. However, dissociation can interrupt this flow. Dissociation is a deeply ingrained, adaptive response to internal experiences that the client feels unable or unwilling to confront in the present.

Where does a client go when they dissociate? It's hard to say definitively. Often, they retreat inward—to a psychological corner or perceived safe zone—where they attempt to shield themselves from perceived harm. What makes this complex is that the part of the self that dissociates may not realize they are safe in the present. Dissociation is typically triggered by the reactivation of past memories and unresolved traumas.

This becomes potentially problematic in EMDR because it obstructs the client's ability to notice and process their internal responses. When this happens, it's necessary to stop the processing and implement grounding skills. While grounding techniques should have already been taught, they must be tailored to each client's specific sensory strengths—olfactory, kinesthetic, visual, or auditory methods that bring the client back to the present.

Sometimes, dissociation is a signal that the therapist has tapped into more of the client's neurological network than the client can handle in that moment. In such cases, it's essential to scale down the material and work with smaller, more manageable fragments of the target.

Dissociation doesn't always look like blankness or withdrawal—it can manifest as heavy rumination. Clients may become stuck trying to understand the trauma, including what happened, why it happened, and how they can address it. In these moments, it's helpful to pause and check in with the client. Ask for specific details to understand better what's surfacing and how to guide the client out of avoidance. Keep in thought that left-brain rumination is a keen way to not feel feelings.

It's also crucial to remember that dissociation is not a voluntary process. It is an automatic, protective strategy—not a conscious choice. Clients aren't choosing to derail the session; instead, their nervous systems are attempting to preserve safety.

If dissociation arises, it does not mean the client cannot do EMDR therapy. It simply means the therapist must modulate or titrate the work, adjusting the intensity, speed, or structure to meet the client where they are. The deeper or more frequent the dissociation, the more likely it is that the client is also dealing with intrusive thoughts, memories, or emotional flashbacks.

When considering the concept of structural dissociation, as discussed by Onno van der Hart, Kathy Steele, and Suzette Boon in their book, *The Haunted Self*, we recognize that dissociation exists on a spectrum. Through deep attunement, therapists must assess the degree of dissociation in the client and adjust their approach accordingly.

For clients with severe dissociation, consider using Ad de Jongh's EMDR 2.0, a modified protocol built around distraction-based processing. For example, engaging the client in unpredictable eye movements, tapping sequences, or cognitive tasks like counting backward while balancing on one foot can provide sufficient distraction to permit safe processing without overwhelming the nervous system.

Finally, when we reflect on the term *dissociation*, we often imagine a client going deep within. But etymologically, dissociation simply means "not associating" with the present. That disconnection can be inward or outward—it may present as zoning out, numbness, or even externalized responses, such as anger, agitation, or oppositional behavior.

Dissociation signals a need to slow down, ground oneself, and titrate the material.

- Use tailored sensory grounding, break targets into fragments, or shift to distraction techniques.
- Understand it's not a failure, but a message from the nervous system.
- Adjust the approach, not the client.

Attunement remains the most critical tool. With presence, patience, and precision, we can safely guide clients back into connection with themselves and the present.

Blocking Beliefs

What are blocking beliefs? They are closely related to negative beliefs, but with one key distinction—they tend to hinder EMDR processing. These beliefs aren't just distortions of self-worth; they act as internal gatekeepers, protecting the client from emotional overwhelm by restricting access to vulnerable or painful material.

In EMDR therapy, effective processing depends on the client's ability to access and activate difficult memories. But if there's a belief such as *"It's not safe to feel,"* the process often stalls. These blocking beliefs can prevent emotional engagement and disrupt the system's capacity to metabolize traumatic memory.

As clinicians, it's essential to recognize that such beliefs often surface not as resistance but as a form of protection. When a client presents with a belief that seems to shut down access to emotional material, the appropriate response is not to push harder, but to explore the issue more deeply. This may include stabilizing the client, building emotional tolerance, or creating internal safety through containment and grounding strategies.

Importantly, a blocking belief does not mean the client is incapable of benefiting from EMDR therapy. Rather, it signals a need for more preparation and resourcing before re-entering the processing phases. These beliefs often reflect gaps in the client's adaptive neural network—the part of the brain responsible for integrating experiences into a coherent, safe narrative.

Blocking beliefs frequently have roots in attachment wounds. Children absorb messages—both spoken and unspoken—from their caregivers and surroundings. Over time, these form coping strategies meant to preserve physical or emotional safety. Some of these become deeply ingrained beliefs that the world, or emotions themselves, are unsafe.

To address blocking beliefs effectively, it's helpful to challenge them from the perspective of an informed, resourced aspect of self, often the adult self. The client may need support in differentiating from the part of themselves that holds the blocking belief, usually a younger or wounded version of self who learned that emotions equaled danger.

The therapeutic goal here is not to eliminate the belief, but to understand and honor its protective intent. By adding positive, adaptive resources, we respect the role that belief once played, while showing the client that there are now other ways to stay safe. This work often involves parts work methodologies, such as Internal Family Systems (IFS) and Ego State Therapy, or other integrative approaches.

It's also important to acknowledge that blocking beliefs can sometimes be blessings in disguise. They have kept the client emotionally and sometimes physically safe. But over time, these beliefs numb all emotions, including joy, love, trust, and connection.

When a client says, *"If I didn't believe this, I could die,"* we must listen closely. This statement isn't a metaphor—it's memory. For many, these beliefs originated in moments of survival. The belief may have made perfect sense in childhood or trauma, but now, in the safety of therapy, it may be time to gently question its relevance and help the client construct a new, adaptive internal truth.

When adult aspects of self become aware of these outdated, protective beliefs, we can invite them into dialogue with the younger parts that still hold the fear. With care, respect, and attunement, we can help clients begin the work of reclaiming their emotional lives without betraying the parts that protected them for so long.

To begin addressing a blocking belief, we can first look at the *anticipated positive belief* about the Self. This belief, however, often feels unreal or unreachable to the client, especially when unresolved trauma is still active in the system. In such cases, we turn to personal resourcing. This involves helping the client recall and connect with moments in their life when they were already embodying the positive belief—times when they *were strong, safe, capable, or loved*, even if only for a moment or in situations that seem small and insignificant.

Once several of these lived experiences are identified, slow bilateral stimulation can be applied to help instill these positive memories as adaptive, internal resources. This creates a corridor for healing, anchoring the client to their capacity for resilience and re-patterning the nervous system's response to vulnerability.

Attachment Repairs

What is attachment?

From conception through early childhood, infants receive information from their caregivers primarily through sensory and somatic channels. Crying is a child's early form of communication, signaling hunger, discomfort, or the need for comfort and reassurance. When those cries are ignored or inconsistently met, the child either escalates the distress or shuts down—an "innie or outie" behavioral response.

This creates what we might call information deficits, which often lead to maladaptive adaptive behaviors. Attachment, by definition, implies connection—something or someone to *hook onto*. But when there's no hook or nothing to hook on to, or if the hook is broken—due to absent, dismissive, or unresponsive caregiving (for possibly all the right reasons)—attachment wounds form. Over time, these wounds often recur, shaping the client's adult relationships and emotional coping mechanisms.

Clients may not recognize these patterns. They may say, *"I had a great childhood,"* but that's a cue, not a conclusion. Gently inquire:

- *"What do you mean by 'great'?"*

This question may reveal the attachment wound narrative. For example:

"We had plenty of money, and my mom had a nanny from day one. When I cried, the nanny brought me to my mom."

This reflects disconnection. The attachment formed with the nanny, not the mother, and the mother might have remained unattuned to the child's needs. Despite material "plenty," there may be an emotional deficit.

In parts work, we can develop nurturing figures to provide emotional attunement to the client's wounded parts. These figures help the client feel sensed, seen, and safe—even if that attunement is being established for the first time in the present.

Somatic Targets in EMDR Therapy

Somatic targets are memories that exist in the body, not in words. These are *implicit memories*—encoded in sensations, whether positive or negative, such as tightness, heat, nausea, or disconnection. Clients may not remember what happened, but their bodies do.

When asked about early memories, a client may say,

"I don't remember, but I get a weird feeling in my stomach."

That's a somatic memory.

As Bessel van der Kolk famously noted, *"The body keeps the score."* These sensations are viable targets, just as real and important as cognitive or narrative memories. The prefrontal cortex may not have been developed enough at the time of trauma to form verbal memory, but the body's memory remains accessible through EMDR.

Use the standard EMDR protocol, adapting your language and approach to meet the client where they are. Ask open-ended, *non-intrusive* questions like:

- *"Did you have a favorite food growing up?"*
- *"Did you have a pet?"*
- *"Did you walk to school or ride a bus?"*

These questions may serve as safe access points—they often bypass resistance and open the door to traumas of omission (what was needed but never received) or traumas of commission (what was done and shouldn't have been done).

Allow clients to name their experience in their own terms. You don't need them to use clinical language or force a narrative that fits the EMDR manual. What matters is that they know what they're noticing.

Sometimes clients use code words—symbols, metaphors, or internal shorthand. That's enough. The unconscious mind knows exactly what it's working on. Our job is to trust that process and remain deeply attuned.

Key Therapeutic Principles

- **Blocking beliefs** can protect clients but may stall EMDR. Work with them, not against them. Resourcing and parts work help soften these barriers.
- **Attachment wounds** often lie beneath current distress. Ask curious, open-ended questions to uncover emotional gaps in "perfect" childhoods.
- **Somatic targets** are legitimate. Trust the body. Use grounding, titration, and slow BLS to assess and process what the client cannot yet name.
- **Client expression matters more than clinical form.** The modality of memory—word, image, sensation, metaphor—does not matter. What matters is that *it's true* for the client.

With patience, attunement, and flexibility, EMDR becomes not just a technique but a deeply reparative experience.

Balancing Presence for Processing

In EMDR therapy, we aim to keep the client with one foot in the present and one foot in the past. This means the client must be grounded enough in the present moment to access and process traumatic content from earlier times, safely. This balance is essential for successful reprocessing.

If a client begins to "fuzz out," dissociate, or seems unable to notice changes between bilateral stimulation sets, it's a clear sign that more preparation might be needed. That preparation may include parts work, grounding skills, visualization exercises, or resource installation—whichever methods are most supportive of the client's ability to maintain dual awareness.

Remember, EMDR therapy is both a standalone and an adjunct modality. Parts work can support EMDR, and EMDR can enrich parts work. The integration of modalities enables a more flexible and client-centered approach. You may notice early signs of protective dissociation during the biopsychosocial phase of treatment—this is often where the seeds of fragmentation and defense structures become visible. These clues are valuable and should not be ignored.

Getting the Correct Belief Structure

In EMDR therapy, cognitions (beliefs) are not just supporting elements—they are the cornerstones of the work. Without a clear, viable belief structure, the neurological network cannot effectively process and integrate the targeted memory.

But which belief matters most?

Let's step back and explore the origins of our beliefs. When a client experiences trauma that overwhelms their capacity to cope, the memory gets stored in a fragmented or maladaptive form. The neurological system then encodes this event with a corresponding meaning about the self. These are not just thoughts—they become deeply held *truths* that shape identity.

To access these beliefs, you can ask the client:

- *"Given all that's happened, what has it made you believe about yourself?"*

If they struggle to answer, redirect the question to a younger part of self:

- *"If this happened to a child, what might that child come to believe about themselves?"*

This question often yields deeper insights. The client's protective parts may still be wary, but their wisdom will emerge when given a compassionate path.

Prioritizing the Positive Cognition

Contrary to what some may assume, a positive belief is more important than a negative one. Why? Because in reprocessing trauma, we are not simply dismantling pain—we are redirecting it into a healthier cognitive corridor. Like a neurological Pac-Man, the positive belief "digests" the harmful material by offering strength, meaning, and stability.

The positive belief must:

- Be about the self only, not others, situations, or outcomes.
- Be grounded in being, not doing.
- Reflect internal strength, not external dependence.

For example:

- *Not: "I am safe because my partner protects me."*
- *Instead: "I am ok, regardless."*
- When forming or refining the positive cognition, try it on.

Ask yourself:

- *"Do the words the client is using make sense in the context of their neurological resilience?"*
- *"Is this belief strong enough to carry the negative memory through processing and integration?"*

If not, slow down and revisit the client's internal truth, not just the aspirational one. You're not looking for an affirmation—they don't need to believe it *yet*—but it must be a belief the system can eventually recognize as *true enough* to process toward.

Kinesthetic Anchors

What are kinesthetic anchors? Remember back when we were little and were given elastic bracelets to snap when we weren't feeling well? That was a kinesthetic anchor—something used to allow the body and brain to alter the response to a stimulus.

When we are installing positive thoughts and feelings, we can use a designated spot on the hand or arm as a sort of "button" for the somatic and cognitive systems to recall a more adaptive stance. This means that we first elicit the positive state and, with slow, short sets of bilateral stimuli, install the feeling sense in the neurological system.

Next, we ask the client to find a minor point—a mole, a knuckle, a brown mark on their hand or arm, or a bony protrusion—

and, when they feel the adaptive feeling, to simply touch the point they have chosen. Then, we ask the client to think of something very mildly intrusive and to focus on the selected point while touching it (i.e., pressing the button). We then ask the client what they experienced and coach them to understand that they can press their feel-adaptive button at any time they wish.

What Was It Like Before?

Sometimes, clients lament the way things were before a trauma occurred. This means they recall what life was like beforehand. Just like with the flash-forward technique—where we ask the client to imagine the future—we can ask them to flash back to a time before the traumatic event.

Trauma alters perception and states of consciousness, and protective mechanisms are often activated. When we ask the client to engage with what it was like before, we are inviting them to recall a time when the trauma was not present. If the client can safely access this without feeling the loss (real or perceived), we can use slow BLS to tap it in, allowing the entire system—thoughts, somatic responses, and emotions—to experience a neutral or improved state.

Keep in mind that pain, both psychological and physical, is protective, and the mind generates protective strategies. When referencing what it was like before, we can guide the client to work with a more neutral state.

Distancing

While some clients can easily connect to their trauma recall, many may not. It can be useful for the clinician to use what we call distancing techniques. One approach might be to suggest that the client observe the part of themselves that has sustained the trauma. From that vantage point, a natural distance exists between the client's present self and their past self.

We can even distance future events for the client. This highlights the difference between objective and subjective experience, creating a buffer for understanding and processing. Depending on when in the client's life the trauma occurred—whether as a young child or older—we can access adaptive strength and apply it to the self-aspect the client wants to work with.

Ask questions like, *"If you were that child, what do you think you might be feeling or experiencing?"* This helps separate the client from the experience just enough to be objective and, possibly, able to step into the experience to adaptively process it.

Installation Processing as an Intervention

In Phase 6 of EMDR therapy, we focus on *installation*. This is where we further install the positive belief as it applies to the target we are processing. But how can we use this in other ways to enhance the adaptive stance the client wants in their daily life?

Installation is done using processing-speed BLS, meaning we are working with the adaptive network to further strengthen its intent. So, why not—when the client is stable and not experiencing negative activation—use this to process other life events that the client identifies as troublesome?

This would look like the following:

- Have the client think of events that are troublesome—this should occur after larger, more overwhelming events have been processed.
- Hold the positive belief and the troublesome event together, and use processing-speed BLS, with SUDs guiding the process until neutrality or an ecologically acceptable SUD level is achieved.
- Have the client hold their hands together to further instill the information into the body.

Ball of String Processing

Sometimes the client is overwhelmed by the number of targets they are holding—too many to name. "This, this, this, and this..."

It's possible to ask the client to imagine a ball of string or elastic bands, each with a different color. This ball of string or bands can metaphorically represent the entirety of events within a particular cluster of targets. A *cluster of targets* refers to multiple different targets that are all related in some way.

For example, a parent who is physically or mentally ill may exhibit frightening behavior toward a child. As an adult, the client may recall many, many times they felt scared. The narrative becomes lengthy, overwhelming, and emotionally engaging—not enjoyable, not beneficial.

When this happens, we can suggest that the client metaphorically construct a ball of string, with each wisp of string representing a target. Once this is visualized, either internally or through drawing, the client can add the negative belief and then begin to process the ball. It is best to start with EMD; if the client is able to work with it, processing can be titrated to either restricted or full EMDR.

Keep in mind that the client must remain grounded in the present to effectively process the ball of string. Processing would then continue as usual using BLS until the SUD of the ball of string comes down to a manageable level or to zero.

Covert Perceptual Targets

Sometimes a target is not concrete. It may not have happened yet, or it may appear in dreams—possibly nightmares. What the mind perceives can be just as real as if it had occurred. The target might be a well-formed thought or a somatic experience.

In any case, we proceed with EMDR processing as though the thought or target actually happened, using the standard protocol. The unconscious mind often creates distractions that surface as symbolic targets, possibly to avoid confronting real-life disturbing situations.

If that happens, simply proceed with processing whatever the client is able to offer.

With children, for instance, they may create scary, imaginary imagery instead of facing something "real." A child might say, "A dragon is going to eat me." We often see effective processing through sand tray therapy or art therapy, where much of the work is metaphorical in nature.

Parts, Aspects of Self, and Jim Knipe's Internal Healing Dialogue (IHD)

Using a parts model, help the client identify internal parts that:

- Are experienced as separate identities
- Are in conflict with each other
- Are inconsistent or incongruent with one another

Steps:

1. Identify a visual or sensory memory that represents the ongoing conflict between the parts.
2. Help the client develop a clear representation of each conflicting part:
   - Notice how each one looks or feels.
   - Notice how old that aspect might be.
   - See those parts in imagination, or use the two-handed interweave technique (Robin Shapiro): place each aspect of self in each hand, or draw ovals on paper.
3. With the client holding in mind the memory or feeling that represents the conflict between the parts, ask one of the internal parts:
   "When you look at that image, what do you experience?"
   - When the client responds, conduct one or more sets of BLS (about 10 laps).
4. Ask the other internal part/aspect/identity/ego state: *"What is your reply to that?"*
   - BLS (about 10 laps).
5. Then, return to the first ego state and ask: *"What is your reply to that?"*

    - Again, follow with BLS (about 10 laps).
6. Repeat this structured back-and-forth:
    - Holding the conflict image in mind
    - Asking for responses
    - Following each response with BLS (about 10 laps)
    - Continue until resolution begins to emerge

Be alert to disturbing realizations or defenses as they arise—these can be targeted as needed.

Note:

- One part may hold intense post-traumatic disturbance, while another may resist facing it.
- The adult part may respond with shame when asked to look at the child part.

Each of these parts or aspects can be acknowledged, worked with, and brought into alignment.

Three-Prong Processing

Once we have finished processing the initial target or targets, we will explore the remaining incidents outlined in the treatment plan. This includes addressing past experiences, present triggers, and anticipated future challenges.

A *future template* is a processing strategy that helps clients imagine an upcoming situation where emotions, sensations, and cognitions might be triggered. We ask the client to hold the situation in mind along with their positive belief, then run a mental "movie" of themselves adaptively managing the situation while using processing-speed bilateral stimulation. This process may be repeated as needed.

The scenarios used should be realistic and relevant. In addition to future templates, we can also work with *future targets*—imagined situations that evoke anxiety or discomfort in the client.

When we're dealing with anxiety-based targets, it's important to remember that anxiety is a referenced trigger from the past, felt in the present, but always projected into a future scenario. So, if necessary, we should address a few future targets to ensure that the neural network is convinced that processing is complete.

It's also important to recognize that *neural network consolidation* may not be achieved in a single session. Full consolidation of past, present, and future elements may take multiple sessions.

Not all clients may want to process every target within the target sequence plan. A question that might arise is: *"What if the client didn't like the processing experience?"* In these cases, we need to attune to the situation. The issue may be that the selected target was not viable or that it was not something the client felt ready to address. Processing may have exceeded the client's *window of tolerance*.

In some cases, the client may fear processing a single incident or may perceive that the act of processing itself is unsafe. When this happens, the client may begin to avoid. At that point, we may consider using Jim Knipe's *Level of Urge to Avoid* protocol—a brief intervention that targets the client's felt sense of how much they want to avoid engaging in processing.

If we still don't understand why the client disliked the experience, we can consider making further adaptations to the way we process targets.

There are two primary approaches to processing:

- **Bottom-up processing** involves starting with smaller, less intense negative targets and gradually working toward building a strong positive neural pathway. It means working from the beginning of the target sequence plan with manageable material.
- **Top-down processing** may be necessary when the client has a complex trauma history, with many interwoven targets. This is like a Jenga tower—processing from the bottom may destabilize the client, potentially leading to decompensation or dissociation due to the sheer weight of what's unresolved.

In such cases, we return to grounding and affect management resources to help the client reestablish presence in the room.

Installation of Safety in the Moment

Jim Knipe

Back of the Head Scale (BHS) Script

The Back of the Head Scale (BHS) is used to assess the extent to which a client is oriented to the present moment, including their awareness of the safety of the current situation. Jim Knipe recommends using the BHS regularly during CIPOS (Constant Installation of Present Orientation and Safety) to monitor for dissociation throughout the procedure. Below is the script provided by Knipe:

The therapist and client participate as follows:

"Think of a line that goes all the way from here..."

(*Extend your arm about 14 inches in front of your face*) *"...running right from my fingers to the back of my head. Now you do the same."*

"Where your hand is now—out in front of you—means that you are completely aware of being present here with me in this room. You can easily listen to what I am saying, and you are not at all distracted by any other thoughts."

"Now move your hand to the back of your head. Let that mean that, even though your eyes are open, in your mind, you are completely in a memory from the past."

(Since even mentioning the trauma memory may cause some loss of present orientation, repeat the description of the scale calmly and matter-of-factly):

"The place out here, with your arm fully extended, means you are completely present. The place at the back of your head means you are fully in the memory. Now, give me an idea of where you are on that line right now."

CIPOS — Constant Installation of Present

Orientation and Safety Script

Jim Knipe

Steps of the CIPOS Procedure:

1. **Provide an Overview**

   Explain the process clearly so the client understands what to expect and can provide informed consent.

2. **Permission**

   Obtain full permission from the client to work on the disturbing memory gradually and safely. Ensure that there is enough time in the session to complete the work, regardless of whether unexpected material arises.

Clients who have dissociated ego states also request permission from any internal parts involved in the memory. If certain parts are unwilling to participate, that is acceptable. However, there must be an agreement from the overall system to allow the memory to be processed.

Suggested language (to be adapted to suit the client):

"I would like to ask all parts of the mind that are involved in this memory for permission to work on this today. Is this okay with all of you?"

Safety

As with any therapeutic intervention, the client must be aware of the *office's objective safety*. If the client appears uncertain about the physical or interpersonal safety in the present moment, this issue should be addressed directly.

Sometimes, through careful observation, inquiry, and discussion, it becomes necessary to help the client recognize that the fears being experienced in the present are actually the result of past events—ones that ended long ago and, often, occurred far away. This *cognitive orientation* to the present reality does not require feelings of safety, but it should be clearly understood on an intellectual level.

If the client expresses uncertainty about the actual safety of your office, any fears or concerns, including transference or countertransference dynamics, should be explored and resolved *before* beginning trauma processing.

If, on the other hand, you're simply unsure about the client's degree of connection to the reality of the safe office, proceed to the next step to clarify their state.

Strengthening Present Orientation

To assess and strengthen the client's sense of being oriented to the present, the therapist may ask a series of simple, concrete questions about the client's current reality in the office. A short set of eye movements or bilateral stimulation should follow each response.

After each client's answer, the therapist says, *"Think of that,"* and initiates a brief set of BLS.

Sample grounding questions include:

- *"Where are you right now, in actual fact?" — "Think of that."*
- *"What do you think of that picture over there?" — "Think of that."*
- *"Can you hear the cars going by outside?" — "Think of that."*
- *"How many tissue boxes do I have in this room?" — "Think of that."*

These questions can be adapted or expanded to match the specific needs of the client. The goal is to strengthen their *sense of being* present.

Another helpful prompt:

- *"What's good about being here right now, instead of somewhere else?"*

Clients often respond with *"I'm comfortable here,"* or *"I know I'm safe here."* Such affirming responses can be strengthened with additional BLS.

- *"Go with that."*

If the client seems puzzled by the simplicity of the questions, explain:

"A firm grounding in present reality is an essential precondition for the use of EMDR to resolve old, disturbing memories. The way EMDR works is: *one foot in the present; one foot in the past.*"

Experiential Grounding Techniques

One especially effective way to help the client anchor in the present is to engage them in a simple sensory or physical task, such as a game of catch:

- "Can you catch this pillow?"
- "Good. Now toss it back."
- *(Repeat 1–10 times, as needed.)*
- "Where are you on the line now?" *(Back of the Head Scale)*

Additional options include:

- "Take a drink of water."
- "Hold this drop of water or an ice cube in your hand."
- "Hum a song and then count to ten."

The game of catch, in particular, appears to reverse derealization in many clients rapidly. Tossing and catching engage the orienting response (OR) as the client tracks the object's trajectory, neurologically anchoring them in the present. According to Wolpe (1958), this action likely reciprocally inhibits the activation of traumatic material, thereby enhancing the client's perception of safety in the present moment.

Other sensory-based grounding techniques—such as water contact or vocal-motor tasks—can similarly promote a shift back to present-time awareness, helping the client feel stabilized and ready to proceed with trauma processing.

The Back of the Head Scale (BHS) and CIPOS *(Jim Knipe)*

Monitoring Presence with the BHS

Through the use of the Back of the Head Scale (BHS), the therapist can assess the effectiveness of CIPOS interventions. This ensures the client remains sufficiently grounded in emotional safety so that trauma reprocessing can occur. The BHS is a reliable tool for confirming that the client remains in the zone of dual attention—that is, maintaining a connection with present safety while accessing traumatic memory material.

By engaging the client in a CIPOS question or action and then asking where they are on the BHS line, the therapist and client can determine whether the client is sufficiently present to begin—or continue—trauma processing.

This process also helps both therapist and client monitor for signs of derealization caused by high levels of intrusive, post-traumatic disturbance. If the client appears to be entering—or is already in—a state of derealization, the therapist should work to reestablish present orientation.

If the client demonstrates sufficient orientation to the present—both over time and in the therapist's judgment—and the client agrees, they may proceed with trauma work.

Beginning Trauma Work Slowly

Once present orientation is well established, you may introduce trauma work gradually:

"In a few moments, would you be willing to close your eyes and go into that memory for just a few seconds—maybe just two seconds? I'll keep track of the time on my watch/phone." (Hold up the watch or phone to make this clear and concrete.)

"Good. Go ahead and do this for [state how many seconds] seconds."

Keep track of the time carefully. This is a carefully controlled dissociative process. Immediately afterward, use soothing, repetitive, and emphatic language to guide the client back to the present:

"Come back into the room now. OK, now come back here. Just open your eyes, find your way back here now. That's right, just open your eyes."

The Importance of Encouragement

At this point, offer supportive but straightforward encouragement:

"Good." or "That's right."

Then resume the CIPOS intervention:

"Where are you right now, in actual fact?"

"Go with that." (*Follow with a short set of BLS.*)

Repeat the process until the client is able to report, using the BHS, that they are once again oriented to the present reality of the therapy room. At that point, step 6 can be repeated.

The rhythm is as follows:

- Pair present safety with BLS
- Then visit the trauma memory for 2–10 seconds *without* BLS
- Return to present safety
- Repeat

Building Resilience Through Repetition

As the process continues, clients develop a growing ability to "stay present." This, in turn, enhances their confidence and emotional control in facing disturbing memories. Over time, this incremental strengthening of dual attention lays the foundation for the use of Standard EMDR Procedures, where bilateral stimulation is directly paired with trauma material.

Parts Work: Aspects of Self

As EMDR therapy evolves, the integration of *parts work* has become a valuable adjunct to standard protocols. Several therapeutic models address this concept, including Internal Family Systems (IFS), Ego State Therapy, and Inner Child Work.

At the core of all these approaches is the understanding that we all have internal aspects of self—*parts* that emerge to promote survival, resilience, and emotional balance, even in distressing circumstances.

When clients develop adaptive mechanisms, they often do so through these parts. Each part fulfills a role that the whole self could not perform under stress. These parts have *benevolent intent*, often protecting the system from further harm or helping it function in the face of adversity.

Richard Schwartz, founder of the Internal Family Systems model, identifies three main types of parts:

1. **Exiles**
   - Holds psychological trauma, often from childhood
   - Carry pain, fear, shame, or rejection
   - They are often pushed away by the system to avoid emotional flooding
2. **Managers**
   - Act preemptively to protect the system from harm
   - Control behavior, thoughts, and interactions to avoid triggering the Exiles
   - May promote perfectionism, people-pleasing, or overfunctioning
3. **Firefighters**
   - Step in reactively when Exiles break through
   - Attempt to extinguish emotional pain quickly and often impulsively

- Behaviors may include substance use, compulsions, aggression, or numbing activities like overworking or binge-watching

IFS posits that beneath all parts is the core Self—a calm, compassionate, curious, and centered presence that can lead the system. The aim of therapy is not to eliminate parts but to build relationships between the Self and each part so that internal harmony is restored.

In IFS, every part—no matter how extreme or dysfunctional its behavior—has a *positive intent*. Healing begins when the Self can listen to and understand the fears, goals, and experiences of each part of the self.

IFS Therapy Goals:

- Access the core Self
- Develop trust and connection between the Self and parts
- Help parts unburden and heal
- Restore balance and inner harmony

Parts work, when combined with EMDR, allows for deeper healing, particularly in clients with complex trauma. It offers a structured yet compassionate lens through which the therapist and client can navigate the rich inner world of protective strategies, unresolved pain, and latent strengths.

Types of Relationships Between Parts

In Internal Family Systems (IFS), three primary types of relationships can exist between parts of the self:

1. **Protection**
   - Managers and Firefighters drive this relationship.
   - Their role is to protect the system from the pain carried by *Exiles*.
   - Managers do this preemptively by controlling behavior and thoughts. Firefighters do it reactively by distracting from emotional overwhelm.

2. **Polarization**
   - Polarization occurs when two parts are locked in conflict, each battling for control of the person's emotional or behavioral response.
   - Each part believes its function is necessary to neutralize or balance the other's extreme behavior.
   - IFS offers specific techniques for identifying, understanding, and working through these internal power struggles.
3. **Alliance**
   - In this dynamic, two different parts collaborate toward a common goal.
   - Though distinct, they operate in tandem to support the same objective within the system.

Integrating IFS with EMDR

IFS can be effectively integrated with EMDR therapy, yielding powerful results, especially in clients with complex trauma, attachment wounds, or dissociation. For clinicians interested in applying this integration skillfully, additional training in IFS is highly recommended.

Ego State Therapy

Ego state therapy is a psychodynamic approach that focuses on resolving inner conflict by working with the distinct parts—or *ego states*—of a person's personality. Each ego state contains its own set of emotions, memories, traits, and coping strategies.

How It Works

- The therapist helps the client identify and connect with their different ego states.
- Drawing from group and family therapy models, the therapist facilitates dialogue and conflict resolution between the ego states.
- The goal is integration—bringing harmony to the system by aligning conflicting states into a cohesive whole.

What It Treats

- Trauma
- PTSD
- Dissociation
- Behavioral and cognitive issues

History

- Ego state therapy was co-developed by **John G. Watkins** and **Helen H. Watkins**.
- Dr. Watkins was a founding member of the International Society for the Study of Dissociation.
- **Robin Shapiro** has also contributed extensively to the clinical application of ego state therapy in her books and teachings.

Like IFS, ego state therapy can be seamlessly woven into EMDR treatment. Clinicians are encouraged to pursue formal training to deepen their skill set in this integrative work.

Developmental Needs Meeting Strategy (DNMS)

Developed by Shirley Jean Schmidt

The Developmental Needs Meeting Strategy (DNMS) is a multidimensional, strengths-based, client-centered approach to ego state therapy, designed to resolve relational and attachment wounds. These may stem from verbal, physical, or sexual abuse as well as neglect, enmeshment, rejection, or chronic misattunement during childhood or adulthood.

What It Does

DNMS uses structured, gentle protocols that:

- Build self-esteem
- Desensitize trauma memories
- Calm hostile introjects
- Reduce internal conflict
- Repair attachment wounds
- Integrate the dissociated parts of the self
- Orient the wounded parts to the present time
- Overcome emotional processing blocks
- Compliment modalities like EMDR
- Reduce unwanted behaviors, beliefs, and emotions

How It Works

- DNMS incorporates alternating bilateral stimulation (similar to EMDR) to facilitate reprocessing of traumatic memories.
- It draws from ego state theory, developmental psychology, attachment theory, self-reparenting, and the neuroscience of mirror neurons.

- Healing occurs through the process of reparenting wounded parts, calming defenses, and integrating them with the client's core self.

What It Treats

DNMS is effective for:

- Complex PTSD
- Depression and anxiety
- Panic and social phobias
- Relationship issues
- Substance abuse
- Eating disorders
- Dissociative disorders
- Safety-sensitive human beings (BPD)
- Sexual abuse and addiction
- Self-injury
- Obsessions and compulsions
- Complicated grief

While DNMS often addresses childhood-origin emotional wounds, it is equally capable of resolving trauma from adulthood.

Each of these approaches—IFS, Ego State Therapy, and DNMS—offers a unique and efficient way to work with complex internal systems. When carefully integrated with EMDR, they can empower clients to reclaim internal harmony, safety, and wholeness.

Future Prong

A quick reminder about the third prong of EMDR therapy: the *future prong*.

Keep in mind that trauma-protective mechanisms are designed to keep our clients safe, and safety is often projected into the future based on past experiences. This is what we call *anxiety*.

Anxiety is a memory—whether real or perceived—felt in the present as a trauma response. It typically refers to the future, anticipating that something painful or threatening may recur. The client's protective system may either shut down or act out in an effort to guard against real or imagined harm.

Because of this, it's essential to understand that therapy may not feel complete until *future templates and targets* are addressed. While reprocessing past events can certainly alleviate the system's burden and provide immediate relief, feelings about the future may linger unless they are explicitly addressed. Completing this third prong is what ensures the client can confidently move forward.

Thoughts and Wisdom

It is of utmost importance to *know, understand, and practice* the basic EMDR protocol as laid out by Francine Shapiro. However, equally vital—if not more so—is the clinician's *attunement* to the client.

Clients come to us with problems, stories, and wounds—but beneath their words lie the *negative thoughts and feelings* that surround the heart. The clinician's curiosity opens the door to understanding these patterns of behavior, which are often the very symptoms of trauma.

When we attune to a client across their lifespan, we begin to notice how trauma affects *thoughts and feelings*. Trauma shuts down the *thinking brain* and activates the *autonomic brain*, which responds reflexively to protect the client, whether or not the danger is real.

Our role is to *educate* clients about their strengths and help them reprocess the events that have caused distress. The human system wants to move forward, and the mind is always doing its best to allow for that progress. The key is having *one foot in the present and one in the past*.

By resourcing our clients *before* setting targets, we help them tap into their own internal strength. That is the art of *attunement*: knowing the protocol and guiding the client toward it gently.

Keep it simple. Be curious, not fearful. And know this: Each person you work with *wants* strength and *has* strength. And so do you.

A Note on Inner Wisdom

When we share our collective knowledge and wisdom with you, the reader, we are also inviting you to *be yourself*. Trust your inner *intuition*.

Most clients already know that their reactions are often not about the current stimulus itself, but rather about a deeper trigger from their past. That's why a current event may not seem significant in reality, yet evoke a powerful traumatic response.

If you've ever found yourself unsure of how to proceed with a complex case, remember: your ability to *tune in* to your client is already at work. Listen not just to what they say, but also to what they do not say. Both are equally important.

When words are absent, and stories cannot be told, assume that the client's nervous system is still telling the story. The way they *feel*, *move*, or *react* is evidence of the unresolved trauma—their *neurological narrative*.

And it may not be about what's happening *right now*. It's what we can call *trauma time*. Your attunement is the capacity to witness these responses without needing logical proof or a formal story.

Trauma rarely makes sense in the moment. It's not always coherent, but it is always real. That's why we must attune to what is being presented—instead of, and in addition to, adhering rigidly to protocol. We must use our senses, our instincts, and our training to adapt the protocol for the good of the client.

This work is *an art*, not just a science. Francine Shapiro gave us the science. We, as clinicians, bring the *art,* maybe not with perfect clarity, but with focus—soft focus.

Sometimes, we can help clients heal without ever hearing the story. We see it in their faces, in their posture, in their somatic signals.

And so we don't always need to stir up painful memories to be effective.

We invite you now to receive this wisdom not just with your mind but with your *knowing*. The fear of failure will never lead us where we want to go. But *curiosity* will. And curiosity is the *cornerstone* of attunement.

Welcome to the part of yourself that already knows—and is brave enough to trust that knowing, whether or not it's ever put into words.

References

Baek, H. J., Kim, J. M., & Lee, H. J. (2018). Effects of trauma-focused therapy on cerebral blood flow in patients with post-traumatic stress disorder: A SPECT study. *Psychiatry Research: Neuroimaging*, 277, 27–33.

Baker, C. (2015). *The Art of the Therapist: Inner Work and Emotional Awareness in Psychotherapy*. New York: Routledge.

Bedi, R. P. (2006). The Role of the Therapeutic Alliance in Psychotherapy with Adolescents. *Journal of Clinical Psychology,* 62(1), 81-92.

Benson, H., & Proctor, W. (2010). *Relaxation Revolution: Enhancing Your Personal Health Through the Science and Practice of Mindfulness.* Harvard Health Publications.

Bowers, J. (2020). *The Nervous System and Foot Sensitivity*. Journal of Bodywork and Movement Therapies, 24(4), 12-19.

Brown, L. S. (2013). *Cultural competence in trauma therapy: Addressing diversity and inclusion*. Routledge.

Brown, R. P., Fridlund, A. J., & Kelsey, E. (2013). *Breathing through the nose: The benefits of nasal breathing for health and well-being*. Journal of Healthcare, 5(2), 121-128.

Cuijpers, P., Karyotaki, E., Weitz, E., Andersson, G., Hollon, S. D., & van Straten, A. (2016). The effects of psychotherapies for major depression in adults on remission, recovery and improvement: A meta-analysis. *Journal of Affective Disorders*, 202, 511-516

Doe, A. B. (2019). Using the 5-4-3-2-1 grounding technique in therapy: Step-by-step instructions. *American Journal of Behavioral Therapy, 12*(4), 300-310. https://doi.org/10.1016/j.ajbt.2019.05.001

Draijer, N. D., & Langeland, W. (2010). Childhood trauma and the development of dissociative symptoms in a clinical sample: The role of trauma and stress. *Journal of Trauma & Dissociation, 11*(2), 143-159. https://doi.org/10.1080/15299730903020004

Fateh, A., Ahmad, S., & Riaz, A. (2017). Neurobiological mechanisms of Eye Movement Desensitization and Reprocessing (EMDR) therapy: A review. *Journal of Neurotherapeutics*, 21(2), 121–129.

Fisher, J. (2017). *The Therapist's Notebook for Integrating Spirituality in Counseling: Homework, Handouts, and Activities for Use in Therapy*. New York: Routledge.

Foa, E. B., Liebowitz, M. R., Kozak, M. J., Davis, R., & Papakostas, G. I. (2010). Randomized, placebo-controlled trial of exposure and ritual prevention, clomipramine, and their combination in the treatment of obsessive-compulsive disorder. *American Journal of Psychiatry*, 167(1), 87-94

Forgash, C. & Knipe, J. (2007). Integrating EMDR and Ego State Treatment for Clients with Trauma Disorders. In C. Forgash, C. and M.Copeley (Eds.) *Healing the heart of trauma and dissociation*. New York: Springer.

Freeman, J., Kessler, J. A., & Koss, M. P. (2022). *The Art and Science of EMDR Therapy*. Journal of Trauma & Dissociation, 23(2), 145-160.

Germer, C. K., & Neff, K. D. (2013). Self-Compassion in Clinical Practice. *Journal of Clinical Psychology*, 69(8), 856-867.

Goleman, D. (1995). Emotional Intelligence: Why It Can Matter More Than IQ. Bantam Books.

Gonzalez, A., Thorne, K., & Tuner, J. (2015). *Using the Therapeutic Relationship in EMDR: Enhancing Treatment Outcomes through Collaboration*. *Journal of EMDR Practice and Research*, 9(3), 141-153.

Gross, J. J., & John, O. P. (2003). Finding meaning in the emotions: An introduction to the special issue on affect and the self. *Journal of Personality and Social Psychology*, 85(1), 1-6.

Hase, M., Hohenshil, T. H., & Voss, E. (2019). *EMDR: A Comprehensive Guide to the Treatment of Trauma*. London: Routledge.

Hase, M., Goldstein, D., & Schmid, K. (2016). Attunement in EMDR: An Adaptive Approach. *Journal of EMDR Practice and Research, 10*(3), 157-167.

Hassett, L. M., & Tully, M. A. (2021). The role of physical activity in mental well-being: A review of the evidence. *International Journal of Environmental Research and Public Health, 18*(9), 4592.

Harris, C., & Caspi, Y. (2010). Cultural considerations in EMDR therapy: A review of the literature. *Journal of EMDR Practice and Research*, 4(2), 78-85. https://doi.org/10.1891/1933-3196.4.2.78

Hart, S. N. (1993). Healing the wounded inner child. New York, NY: HarperOne.

Hensley, S. (2020). *EMDR therapy: A comprehensive guide*. New York: Therapy Press.

Hill, J. K., Litz, B. T., & Hetrick, S. E. (2020). Efficacy of EMDR for PTSD: A meta-analysis. *Journal of Traumatic Stress*, 33(1), 1-10

Hintermair, M. (2011). "And the Art of Human Connection". *Journal of EMDR Practice and Research*, 5(4), 193-202.

Hodge, F., & Nadir, A. (2018). Cultural competence in trauma therapy: Embracing diversity in clinical practice. *Trauma, Violence, & Abuse*, 19(2), 123–134.

Hofmann, S. G., Asnaani, A., Vonk, I. J. J., Sawyer, A. T., & Fang, A. (2012). The Efficacy of Cognitive Behavioral Therapy: A Review of Meta-analyses. *Cognitive Therapy and Research*, 36(5), 427-440.

Hofmann, S. G., Asnaani, A., Vonk, I. J. J., Sawyer, A. T., & Fang, A. (2012). "The Efficacy of Cognitive Behavioral Therapy: A Practice-Friendly Meta-Analysis." *American Psychologist*, 67(1), 43-55.

Hogberg, B., Berrios, R., & Elklit, A. (2020). Neuroimaging in EMDR: A Review of the Latest Findings. *Journal of EMDR Practice and Research*, 14(1), 27-40.

Jarero, I. N., & Artigas, L. (2024). The EMDR Therapy Butterfly Hug Method for Self-Administered Bilateral Stimulation: Technical Report. May 2024.

Kabat-Zinn, J. (2003). Mindfulness-based interventions in context: Past, present, and future. Clinical Psychology: Science and Practice, 10(2), 144-156.

Kox, M., van Eijk, L. T., Zwaag, J., van den Wildenberg, J., Sweep, F. C., van der Hoeven, J. G., ... & Pickkers, P. (2014). *Voluntary activation of the sympathetic nervous system and attenuation of the innate immune response in humans*. Proceedings of the National Academy of Sciences, 111(20), 7379-7384.

Knipe, J. (2015) *EMDR Toolbox: Theory and Treatment of Complex PTSD and Dissociation*. (pp 195-204). New York: Springer Publishing Company.

Knipe, J. (2008). The CIPOS method-procedures to Therapeutically reduce dissociative processes while preserving emotional safety. Master class at the EMDR European Conference, London.

Kira, I. A., Ashby, J. S., Lewandowski, L., & Alhussain, A. (2014). *Cultural competence in trauma therapy: Addressing diversity and inclusion*. Journal of Trauma & Dissociation, 15(3), 283–298.

Kivlighan, D. M., & Tully, L. A. (2023). *Personalized Therapy: Tailoring Therapeutic Approaches to Enhance Client Outcomes*. Journal of Counseling Psychology, 70(2), 215-229.

Laganiere, C., & Bouchard, R. (2019). Grounding techniques: Applications in trauma-informed care. *Journal of Trauma & Dissociation*, 20(5), 529-548. https://doi.org/10.1080/15299732.2019.1576395

Lee, K. J., & Cuijpers, P. (2013). Emotional and cognitive processing in EMDR: A critical review. *Journal of EMDR Practice and Research*, 7(2), 60-63.

Leeds, A. M. (2016). *EMDR: A comprehensive guide to a powerful new therapy for trauma*. Wiley.

Levine, P. A. (1997). *Waking the tiger: Healing trauma: The innate capacity to transform overwhelming experiences*. North Atlantic Books.

Levy, S., & Orlans, V. (2016). *The Handbook of Therapeutic Attachment: Special Issues in Psychotherapy*. Routledge.

Luber, M., & Shapiro, F. (2003). EMDR Supervision: A Training Program. *Journal of EMDR Practice and Research*, 1(4), 307-315.

Luber, B., & Lisanby, S. H. (2014). Enhancing human learning, memory, and cognitive performance with transcranial magnetic stimulation (TMS). *NeuroImage*, 85, 961–970.

Lutz, A. (2015). Sleep and brain function. In R. R. Bootzin & P. D. O'Connor (Eds.), Behavioral treatment for sleep disorders: A comprehensive primer (pp. 131-146). American Psychological Association.

Mackay, C. E., Kox, M., van der Hoeven, J. G., Pickkers, P., & van der Hoeven, J. G. (2012). *Voluntary suppression of physiological responses to stress*. Journal of Applied Physiology, 113(10), 1555-1562.

Macksoud, M. S., & Aber, J. L. (1996). The Impact of Exposure to War on Children: An Unanswered Question. *Journal of Traumatic Stress*, 9(2), 241-257.

Maxfield, L., & Hyer, L. (2002). *EMDR in the treatment of complex trauma: Targeting the developmental needs of clients*. Journal of EMDR Practice and Research, 1(2), 93–109. https://doi.org/10.1891/1933-3196.1.2.93

McLeod, J. (2015). *An Introduction to Counselling* (5th ed.). Open University Press.

Mender, B. (2020). Creating Safety in the Therapeutic Space: A Framework for Trauma-Informed Care. *Psychological Trauma: Theory, Research, Practice, and Policy*, 12(1), 81-88.

Meyer, A., & Turner, H. (2023). *The Role of Empathy in Psychotherapy: Enhancing Trust and Improving Outcomes*. Journal of Counseling Psychology, 70(2), 155-167.

Miller, W. R., & Rollnick, S. (2023). *Motivational Interviewing: Helping People Change* (4th ed.). Guilford Press.

Müller, I., et al. (2018). The effects of eye movement desensitization and reprocessing therapy on functioning and quality of life in PTSD patients: a randomized controlled trial. *European Journal of Psychotraumatology*, 9(1)

Nascimento, D. S., Barros, A. F., & Pacheco, R. W. (2019). *The effects of breathing techniques on mental health outcomes: A systematic review*. Journal of Mental Health Research, 29(3), 234-244.

Nienhuis, J,B., Owen J., Valentine, J, C., Winkeljohn Black, S., Halford, T,C., Parazak S,E., Budge, S., & Hilsenroth, M. (2018). *Therapeutic alliance, empathy, and genuineness in individual adult psychotherapy: A meta-analytic review*. Psychotherapy Research. 28(4):593-605. http://doi: 10.1080/10503307.2016.1204023

Norcross, J. C., & Lambert, M. J. (2018). *The Therapeutic Alliance: An Evidence-Based Guide to Practice*. Psychotherapy, 55(4), 392-404.

Norcross, J. C. (2011). *Psychotherapy relationships that work: Evidence-based responsiveness.* Oxford University Press.

Norcross, J. C. (2011). "The Therapeutic Relationship: An Evolutionary Perspective." In J. C. Norcross (Ed.), *Psychotherapy relationships that work: Evidence-based responsiveness* (pp. 26-39). Oxford University Press.

Ogden, P., Minton, K., & Pain, C. (2006). *Sensorimotor Psychotherapy: Interventions for Trauma and Attachment*. New York: Norton & Company.

Ogden, P., & Minton, K. (2000). *Sensorimotor Psychotherapy: Interventions for Trauma and Abuse*. New York: Norton & Company.

Ogden, P., & Fisher, J. (2015). *Sensorimotor Psychotherapy: Interventions for Trauma and Attachment*. W. W. Norton & Company.

Pagani, M., et al. (2018). "Functional neuroimaging of eye movement desensitization and reprocessing therapy in patients with post-traumatic stress disorder: an exploratory study." *Psychological Trauma: Theory, Research, Practice, and Policy*, 10(5), 539-547.

Paulson, S., & Spear Chief, S. (2019). Integrating cultural awareness into EMDR therapy: Enhancing cultural sensitivity for better therapeutic outcomes. *Journal of Trauma & Dissociation*, 20(3), 317–332.

Paulson, S., & Spear Chief, S. (2020). Challenges and barriers in cross-cultural EMDR practice: Attuning to diverse cultural expressions of trauma. *Trauma, Violence, & Abuse*, 21(2), 334–347.

Paulson, S., & Spear Chief, S. (2022). The effectiveness of culturally adapted EMDR interventions: Enhancing client engagement and symptom reduction. *Journal of Trauma Therapy, 15*(3), 123-135.

Perry, B. D. (2009). "The Neurosequential Model of Therapeutics." *Child Trauma Academy*. Retrieved from Child Trauma Academy Website.

Saj, C., & Mete, R. (2025). The IDEA Framework: Integrating Positive Psychology, Yoga, Hypnotherapy, and Bilateral Stimulation for Safety, Stabilization, and Healing of Well-Being. *International Journal of Positivity & Well-Being, 3*(1). https://doi.org/10.61518/ijpw-111

Safran, J. D., & Muran, J. C. (2000). *Negotiating the Therapeutic Alliance: A Relational Treatment Guide*. New York: Guilford Press.

Scaer, R. C. (2005). Trauma spectrum. New York, NY: W.W. Norton & Company.

Schmidt, S. J. (n.d.). The DNMS: What it is and how it works.

Schore, A. N. (2003). Affect regulation and the origin of the self: The neurobiology of emotional development. Norton Series on Interpersonal Neurobiology. Norton.

Shapiro, F. (2001). *Eye movement desensitization and reprocessing: Basic principles, protocols, and procedures*. Guilford Press.

Shapiro, F. (2014). *Eye Movement Desensitization and Reprocessing (EMDR) Therapy: Basic Principles, Protocols, and Procedures* (2nd ed.). Guilford Press.

Shapiro, F. (2014). *EMDR Therapy: An Integrative Approach to Treating Trauma and Other Disorders*. New York: Guilford Press.

Shapiro, F. (2017). *Eye Movement Desensitization and Reprocessing: Basic Principles, Protocols, and Procedures*. New York: Guilford Press.

Shapiro, F. (2018). *Eye Movement Desensitization and Reprocessing (EMDR) Therapy: Basic Principles, Protocols, and Procedures* (3rd ed.). Guilford Publications

Shapiro, Robin. (2016) Easy Ego State Intervention W.W. Norton & Company

Siegel, D. J. (2010). *The Mindful Therapist: A Clinician's Guide to Mindsight and Neural Integration*. W. W. Norton & Company.

Siegel, D. J. (1999). *The Developing Mind: Toward a Neurobiology of Interpersonal Experience.* New York: Guilford Press.

Solomon, R. M., & Rothbaum, B. O. (2004). EMDR and the Adaptive Information Processing Model: Integrating Memory Processing in the Treatment of Trauma. *Journal of Clinical Psychology*, 60(3), 333-346.

Spear Chief, S. (2017). *Cultural awareness and sensitivity in therapy: Enhancing trust and engagement with Indigenous and marginalized communities.*

Stein, M. B., Hultman, C. M., & Kivlighan, D. M. (2012). Interpersonal Processes in TM-EMDR: Developing and Testing a Framework for Safe and Effective Trauma Therapy. *Journal of Traumatic Stress*, 25(2), 169-178.

Stern, D. N. (1985). The Interpersonal World of the Infant. Basic Books.

Sweeney, A., & Myers, L. (2023). *Creating Safe Spaces: The Impact of Supportive Environments on Client Engagement in Therapy*. Counselling Psychology Review, 38(1), 45-60.

Trevarthen, C. (2011). The foundations of emotional communication: Infants' intersubjectivity. The Interpersonal Neurobiology of Play, 29-52.

Walker, M. P. (2017). *Why We Sleep: Unlocking the Power of Sleep and Dreams*. Scribner.

Watkins, C. E., & Riggs, S. A. (2023). *Advancing Counseling Theory: The Impact of Depth and Nuance on Therapeutic Effectiveness*. Journal of Counseling & Development, 101(4), 486-497.

Watts, B. V., Lawson, W., Seko, K., & Keller, A. (2013). A systematic review of the evidence for the efficacy of EMDR in the treatment of PTSD. *Psychological Trauma: Theory, Research, Practice, and Policy*, 5(6), 242-247.

Valiente, C. (2018). Developing Therapeutic Relationships: Practical Strategies for Building Trust with Clients. *Journal of Counseling Psychology*, 65(1), 50-58.

Van der Kolk, B. A. (2014). *The Body Keeps the Score: Brain, Mind, and Body in the Healing of Trauma*. New York: Penguin Books.

Young, K. L., Klosko, J. S., & Weishaar, M. E. (2003). Schema therapy: A practitioners' guide. Guilford Press.

Zimmerman, Thomas. (2024) EMDR With Complex Trauma. EMDR Training Collaborative

www.ingramcontent.com/pod-product-compliance
Lightning Source LLC
LaVergne TN
LVHW050913210926
848482LV00012B/421